Assessing hypertension control and management

2

WHO Library Cataloguing in Publication Data

Assessing hypertension control and management :
hypertension management audit project : a WHO/WHL
study / edited by T. Strasser and L. Wilhelmsen

(WHO regional publications. European series ; No. 47)

1.Hypertension – prevention & control 2.Evaluation
3.Europe I.Strasser, T. II.Wilhelmsen, L. III.World
Hypertension League IV.Series

ISBN 92 890 1310 9 (NLM Classification: WG 340)
ISSN 0378-2255

Cover design based on a poster entitled "Don't beat your heart beat",
entered in the 1991 WHL International Art Competition
by Galit Aka-Maurer, Israel.

World Health Organization
Regional Office for Europe
Copenhagen

World Hypertension League
Geneva

Assessing hypertension control and management

Hypertension Management Audit Project: a WHO/WHL study

Edited by

T. Strasser and L. Wilhelmsen

WHO Regional Publications, European Series, No. 47

ICP/CVD 122
Text editing by Pamela M. Charlton

ISBN 92 890 1310 9
ISSN 0378-2255

CONTENTS

FOREWORD

With a prevalence of up to 30% in certain populations and with its serious effects on health, arterial hypertension is a major public health problem in the European Region. Through its cardiovascular disease programme, the Regional Office has turned increasing attention to the management of hypertension, which will play an important part in the achievement of target 9 of the European health for all policy, to reduce mortality from diseases of the circulatory system by 15%. In 1983, the Office launched the European Health Care Related Hypertension Research Action Programme (HYRAP) and designated the Department of Medicine, Östra Hospital, Gothenburg, Sweden, a WHO collaborating centre to coordinate it.

HYRAP included several activities, but the project to assess the levels and quality of the management of hypertension in selected European countries was one of the first. Best known as the Hypertension Management Audit Project, it began in 1983 and became the mainstay of HYRAP. A few years later the World Hypertension League, a nongovernmental organization in official relations with WHO, joined the project, offering technical, organizational and financial input. This collaboration has been an excellent example of cooperation of this kind. I would particularly like to thank the editors of this book, Dr T. Strasser of the World Hypertension League and Dr L. Wilhelmsen of the Gothenburg collaborating centre, for so expertly consolidating the results of the surveys reported in this book, as well as Dr A. Shatchkute, Regional Adviser for Chronic Diseases, for guiding the entire project with such a sure hand.

The lessons to be learnt from the results of the Hypertension Management Audit Project, as described in this volume, are important and numerous. The ultimate message, however, may be summed up in just a few words: the transfer from the theory to the practice of health care needs to be improved. One way is to pinpoint the deficiencies and difficulties found in the care given to people with hypertension. I am confident that, by doing so, the present volume will help bridge some gaps between knowledge and implementation. It will also be very important in the design of better strategies to reduce the problem of stroke in the European Region, a project currently being developed in the Regional Office.

J.E. Asvall
WHO Regional Director for Europe

ACKNOWLEDGEMENTS

The editors wish to express their appreciation to the hard-working investigators who did all the work in the field.

The World Hypertension League acknowledges with sincere thanks a grant received from Boehringer Ingelheim, making the League's participation in this project possible.

CONTRIBUTORS

Editors

T. Strasser, World Hypertension League, Geneva, Switzerland

L. Wilhelmsen, Department of Medicine, Östra Hospital, Gothenburg, Sweden

Principal investigators

R. Accetto, Clinic for Hypertension, University Clinic for Internal Medicine Dr P. Držaja, Ljubljana, Slovenia

E. Apetrei, Centre of Cardiology, Fundeni Clinical Hospital, Bucharest, Romania

B. Bella, National Institute of Pharmacy, Budapest, Hungary

L. Bregman, Department of Medicine B and Clinic for Prevention of Cardiovascular Diseases, Barzilai Medical Centre, Ashkelon, Israel

E. Brenner, Community Health and Tropical Medicine Unit, Institute of Social and Preventive Medicine, University of Geneva, Switzerland

G. Calangiu, Cardiology Department, Slatina Hospital, Romania

V. Canonico, Institute of Internal Medicine, Cardiology and Cardiovascular Surgery, Faculty of Medicine and Surgery, University of Naples, Italy

C. Carp, Centre of Cardiology, Fundeni Clinical Hospital, Bucharest, Romania

B. Cibič, Clinic for Hypertension, University Clinic for Internal Medicine Dr P. Držaja, Ljubljana, Slovenia

I. Coman, Centre of Cardiology, Fundeni Clinical Hospital, Bucharest, Romania

I. David, Cardiology Department, Slatina Hospital, Romania

J. Dobovišek, Clinic for Hypertension, University Clinic for Internal Medicine Dr P. Držaja, Ljubljana, Slovenia

P. Dolenc, Clinic for Hypertension, University Clinic for Internal Medicine Dr P. Držaja, Ljubljana, Slovenia

J. Duba, National Institute of Cardiology, Budapest, Hungary

A. Döring, GSF-Institute for Epidemiology, Neuherberg, Germany

D. Enachescu, Institute of Medicine and Pharmacy, Department of Health, Bucharest, Romania

F. Endrényi, National Institute of Pharmacy, Budapest, Hungary

L. Forgione, Institute of Internal Medicine, Cardiology and Cardiovascular Surgery, Faculty of Medicine and Surgery, University of Naples, Italy

A. Füller, IPG Institute for Prevention and Health Research, Heidelberg, Germany

C. Ginghina, Centre of Cardiology, Fundeni Clinical Hospital, Bucharest, Romania

H.-W. Hense, GSF-Institute for Epidemiology, Neuherberg, Germany

U. Härtel, GSF-Institute for Epidemiology, Neuherberg, Germany

M. Jakovljević, Institute of Social Medicine, Medical Faculty, University of Novi Sad, Yugoslavia (Serbia & Montenegro)

P. Jezeršek, Clinic for Hypertension, University Clinic for Internal Medicine Dr P. Držaja, Ljubljana, Slovenia

U. Keil, GSF-Institute for Epidemiology, Neuherberg and Department of Social Medicine and Epidemiology, Ruhr University Bochum, Germany

E. Klier, Department of Medicine B and Clinic for Prevention of Cardiovascular Diseases, Barzilai Medical Centre, Ashkelon, Israel

M. Klier, Department of Medicine B and Clinic for Prevention of Cardiovascular Diseases, Barzilai Medical Centre, Ashkelon, Israel

B. Kolšek, Clinic for Hypertension, University Clinic for Internal Medicine Dr P. Držaja, Ljubljana, Slovenia

Z. Kralj, Clinic for Hypertension, University Clinic for Internal Medicine Dr P. Držaja, Ljubljana, Slovenia

A. Laaser, IPG Institute for Prevention and Health Research, Heidelberg, Germany

Z. Lapanja, Clinic for Hypertension, University Clinic for Internal Medicine Dr P. Držaja, Ljubljana, Slovenia

A. Laszt, Department of Medicine B and Clinic for Prevention of Cardiovascular Diseases, Barzilai Medical Centre, Ashkelon, Israel

M. Mihelič-Brčič, Clinic for Hypertension, University Clinic for Internal Medicine Dr P. Držaja, Ljubljana, Slovenia

J. Mishal, Department of Medicine B and Clinic for Prevention of Cardiovascular Diseases, Barzilai Medical Centre, Ashkelon, Israel

G. Nandris, Cardiology Department, Sibiu Hospital, Romania

S. Oren, Department of Medicine B and Clinic for Prevention of Cardiovascular Diseases, Barzilai Medical Centre, Ashkelon, Israel

J. Petrin, Clinic for Hypertension, University Clinic for Internal Medicine Dr P. Držaja, Ljubljana, Slovenia

G. Pfaff, German Institute for Hypertension Research, Heidelberg, Germany

D. Pinkesfeld, Department of Medicine B and Clinic for Prevention of Cardiovascular Diseases, Barzilai Medical Centre, Ashkelon, Israel

O. Pirc-Čerček, Clinic for Hypertension, University Clinic for Internal Medicine Dr P. Držaja, Ljubljana, Slovenia

M. Planojević, Communal Institute of Health Protection, City of Novi Sad, Yugoslavia (Serbia & Montenegro)

E. Rab, National Institute of Pharmacy, Budapest, Hungary

F. Rengo, Institute of Internal Medicine, Cardiology and Cardiovascular Surgery, Faculty of Medicine and Surgery, University of Naples, Italy

A. Rougemont, Community Health and Tropical Medicine Unit, Institute of Social and Preventive Medicine, University of Geneva, Switzerland

A. Sabo, Institute of Pharmacology, Medical Faculty, University of Novi Sad, Yugoslavia (Serbia & Montenegro)

V. Schumann, IPG Institute for Prevention and Health Research, Heidelberg, Germany

M. Siegel, IPG Institute for Prevention and Health Research, Heidelberg, Germany

A. Spelsberg, Department of Social Medicine and Epidemiology, Ruhr University Bochum, Germany

M. Stanulović, Institute of Pharmacology, Medical Faculty, University of Novi Sad, Yugoslavia (Serbia & Montenegro)

J. Stieber, GSF-Institute for Epidemiology, Neuherberg, Germany

I. Stoian, Centre of Cardiology, Fundeni Clinical Hospital, Bucharest, Romania

M. Torner i Soler, Advisory Council on Arterial Hypertension in Catalonia, Barcelona, Spain

E. Török, National Institute of Cardiology, Budapest, Hungary

L. La Vecchia, Division of Clinical Cardiology, Local Health Unit No. 8, University of Verona, Vicenza, Italy

M. Vincenzi, Division of Clinical Cardiology, Local Health Unit No. 8, University of Verona, Vicenza, Italy

R.J. Viskoper, Department of Medicine B and Clinic for Prevention of Cardiovascular Diseases, Barzilai Medical Centre, Ashkelon, Israel

S.K. Weiland, Department of Social Medicine and Epidemiology, Ruhr University Bochum, Germany

L. Zaletel-Kragelj, Institute for Biomedical Informatics, Medical School Ljubljana, Slovenia

A. Žemva, Clinic for Hypertension, University Clinic for Internal Medicine Dr P. Držaja, Ljubljana, Slovenia

WHO Regional Office for Europe

V. Zaitsev, formerly Regional Officer for Chronic Diseases

A. Shatchkute, Regional Adviser for Chronic Diseases

P. Charlton, Editor, Publications

SUMMARY

Five approaches were taken to assess hypertension control in various European populations, including one in Israel.

1. The population approach aims to assess the basic indicators of awareness of hypertension in the community: i.e. the proportion of undiagnosed and untreated, or overdiagnosed and possibly unnecessarily treated hypertensive patients.

2. The patient approach concerns patients with an established diagnosis of hypertension. The procedure includes a medical audit of the quality of care they are receiving, on the basis of medical records combined with re-examinations of patients.

3. The consumer approach is an attempt to assess the patients' mood, their readiness to follow advice and their possible complaints about the care they are receiving.

4. The physician approach aims at assessing the knowledge and attitudes of physicians who are involved in the control of hypertension.

5. The drug utilization approach uses established methods of drug utilization studies to assess the volume of antihypertensive drug prescriptions.

Participating centres could take part in all, some or only one of the five approaches.

A total of seven countries in the European Region of WHO were involved. The total of the surveyed population groups exceeded 150 000 individuals and the random samples examined included just over 39 000 men and women. Participation rates ranged from 69% (random samples) to 100% (industrial populations).

The prevalence of confirmed hypertension varies widely; it is considerably lower in the industrial populations (5 – 15%), probably due to selection during recruitment for employment. In the general population samples (age 35 – 64), prevalence rates from about 20% up to 27% were found.

The proportion of newly discovered hypertension varies from 17% to 34%, thus showing an improvement in detection of hypertension as compared with reports from the beginning of the 1970s. The proportion of previously known but untreated hypertensives varies from 22% to 38%, with the exception of the special industrial workers in Romania, where all hypertensives were reported to be under treatment. On average, however, only 29% of all confirmed hypertensives have attained normal blood pressure levels. Thus, an average of 46% of confirmed hypertensives are being treated inadequately.

Diuretics are the leading drug family followed by beta-blockers. Calcium antagonists are given in 3 – 15% of patients and the use of ACE inhibitors varies considerably between countries.

The work-up for hypertensive patients varies considerably in the four centres where it was assessed. The use of body weight measurements ranges from 35% to 96%, chest X-rays from 43% to 92%, eye-ground examinations from 11% to 70%, serum cholesterol measurements from 27% to 92%, and serum potassium measurements from 0% to 59%. By contrast, information on alcohol intake is solicited in 58% of patients at most.

The results of the consumer inquiry show considerable differences between centres. These differences are not necessarily related to the health care *per se*, and could be due to cultural differences between various countries and societies.

Eight physician inquiries were carried out on a sample of 4830 physicians taken from a total of 8281. The overall response rate was slightly over 50%.

The use of aneroid sphygmomanometers is still widespread. A surprising number of physicians report using Korotkoff IV sound; most round off readings to the nearest 5 mmHg, while 3 – 26% admit rounding up to 10 mmHg.

While in all centres most physicians declare starting treatment at 160 mmHg systolic pressure, diastolic cut-off values are given as 95 – 100 mmHg.

Most physicians in most centres ascribe high importance to non-drug treatment and risk factor control, but when cross-checked with information obtained from the patient survey, their actions are less impressive.

In general, more physicians report the need for certain diagnostic methods than can, in fact, be found carrying them out in the patient records.

Information on advances in the management of hypertension seems to reach physicians mostly through medical journals, while other information sources vary greatly.

The process evaluation used in this project has produced a great number of relevant indicators of the quality of antihypertensive management. These are the proportion of awareness of hypertension in the population, the percentage of missed appointments, the distribution of therapeutic attitudes among physicians and the structure of drug prescribing. This project is one of the first to report on patients' satisfaction with the therapy used to manage hypertension. The varied results indicate that much more attention should be paid to this component of hypertension management. Physicians need more formal training in this domain. This project has also shown, however, that new methods are needed to influence physicians' acceptance of and compliance with recommendations for the work-up and management of hypertensive patients.

PART I

OVERVIEW

I

INTRODUCTION

L. Wilhelmsen & T. Strasser

The history of hypertension control can be divided into several periods. Up to the early 1950s, attention focused on severe, mostly intractable cases of hypertension with limited, if any, opportunities for effective treatment. Attempts such as lumbar sympathectomy (Smithwick's operation) are now historical curiosa.

The modern era of hypertension control began at the end of the 1950s with the introduction of the first generation of effective antihypertensive drugs (ganglion blockers, rauwolfia, hydrochlorothiazide). Simultaneously, epidemiologists started to realize the paramount public health importance of elevated blood pressure, the 1959 report of the Society of Actuaries *(1)* having demonstrated the close association of blood pressure values with mortality in the long-term observations of more than five million life insurance policies.

By the early 1970s, facilitated by increasing epidemiological evidence (such as the Framingham study) and the availability of second generation antihypertensive drugs, the crucial importance of moderate and mild hypertension as a risk factor for coronary and cerebrovascular disease and of its treatment came to the fore. This period is characterized by the introduction of cardiovascular and hypertension community control programmes (see *2*) and by the birth, in increasing numbers, of trials of therapy for mild hypertension *(3)*. Stimulated by the results of the trials and of pharmaceutical research, the newer, second generation antihypertensive drugs were developed. The drug treatment of lesser blood pressure elevations became increasingly frequent; around the same time, concern began to grow about the economic aspects of policies for the management of hypertension *(4)*.

The 1980s saw the birth of third generation drugs; the high community attributable risk of mild hypertension *(5)* and the central place of mild hypertension *(6)* were realized. Community programmes proved to be effective *(7)*. The WHO Regional Office for Europe designated hypertension as one of its priorities, and started its Health Care Related Hypertension Research Action Programme (HYRAP) in 1983.

At this stage, it became evident that despite the intensive efforts to implement hypertension control, little was known about how far various recommendations were in fact being followed in the population. Systematic analyses of the practice of hypertension control in populations were missing. Feedback was needed from the field. The present project was therefore developed during 1983 – 1985 to assess the levels of hypertension control in various European populations.

References

1. *Build and blood pressure study*. Chicago, Society of Actuaries, 1959.
2. Strasser, T. Community control of hypertension – international activities. *Health services reports*, **88**: 387 – 390 (1973).
3. WHO/ISH Mild Hypertension Liaison Committee. Trials of the treatment of mild hypertension. An interim analysis. *Lancet*, **1**: 149 – 156 (1982).
4. Weinstein, M.C. & Stason, W.B. *Hypertension: a policy perspective*. Cambridge, MA, Harvard University Press, 1976.
5. *Hypertension related to health care – research priorities*: report on a WHO Consultation. Copenhagen, WHO Regional Office for Europe, 1980 (EURO Reports and Studies, No. 32).
6. Gross, F. & Strasser, T., ed. *Mild hypertension – recent advances*. New York, Raven Press, 1983.
7. Ambrosio, G.B. et al. Effects of interventions on community awareness and treatment of hypertension: results of a WHO Study. *Bulletin of the World Health Organization*, **66**: 107 – 113 (1988).

2

OBJECTIVES, METHODS AND PHILOSOPHY OF THE PROJECT

T. Strasser & L. Wilhelmsen

The control of hypertension, like disease control or health promotion in general, is a complex, multidimensional process. The immediate objective of the project was to assess by simple methods the levels of control of hypertension achieved in various populations. This was to be complemented by the collection of information about various elements of the process of hypertension control. The emphasis was on making the project both simple and multidimensional. Simplicity was needed to offer a readily feasible, realistic project to centres with limited resources and modest epidemiological expertise. But the idea was that, by combining simple individual approaches together, the centres would be able to assess this complex matter in a comprehensive way. Five approaches were chosen as a means of assessing hypertension control in the community (Fig. 1).

1. The population approach comprises a "classical" epidemiological survey of a probability sample of a population: in this case, a community survey. Its aims are to assess the basic indicators of awareness of hypertension in the community, such as the proportion of undiagnosed and untreated or, for that matter, overdiagnosed and possibly unnecessarily treated hypertensive patients. (See Fig. 1 in Annex 1).

2. In the patient approach, a sample of patients with the established diagnosis of hypertension is selected, and their case histories are reviewed by a small committee of investigators. This patient survey includes a medical audit in the strict sense of the term, a "retrospective assessment of the quality of care on the basis of medical records" *(1)*, combined with re-examinations of the patient. A flowchart of the procedures used in the survey is given in Fig. 1, 2 and 3 of the protocol (see Annex 1). The WHO/ISH (International Society of Hypertension) guidelines for the management of mild hypertension *(2)* were selected as the standard of adequate treatment, with which the actual management of the audited cases had to be compared.

3. In the consumer approach, patients are the consumers of medical care, the clients of physicians. Their perceptions and satisfaction are an

Fig. 1. Model of the five approaches

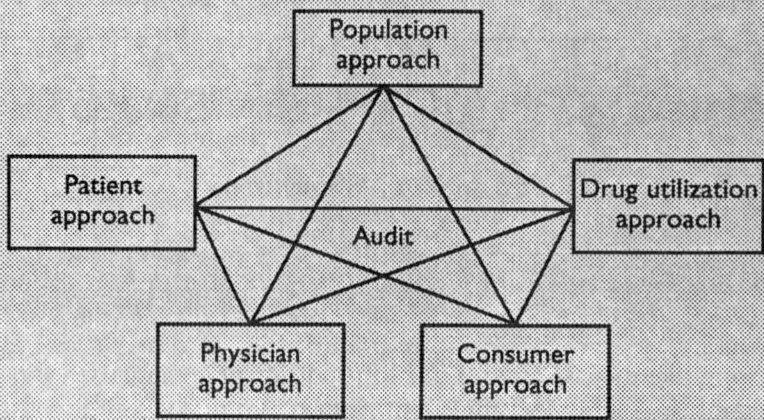

important indicator of certain aspects of the complex process of hypertension control. The consumer inquiry is an attempt to assess the clients' mood, their readiness to follow advice, and their possible complaints about the care received.

4. The physician approach consists of a physician inquiry to assess the knowledge and attitudes of physicians who are involved in the control of hypertension. To this effect a questionnaire is addressed to a sample of general practitioners and internists (see Annex 1). Obviously, the replies are limited to knowledge and attitudes; in all likelihood they do not measure what physicians are in fact doing, but describe rather what they think they ought to do. Still, these "self portraits" of physicians are valuable in the sense that actual behaviour is unlikely to be better than the ideas and intentions of the respondents.

5. Finally, the drug utilization approach uses the established methods of drug utilization studies to assess the volume of antihypertensive drug prescriptions in defined daily doses, related to the number of inhabitants and the prevalence of hypertension. It also assesses the structure of drug utilization. Both amount and structure are valuable health care indices, which may complement the information received from the epidemiological and clinical approaches.

The participating centres were invited to take all five approaches or, if they felt this was beyond their capacity, to select those approaches that seemed to be feasible, in the local circumstances. The information derived from any single approach was expected to be meaningful although, of course, the approaches were complementary to each other, each approach being designed to assess one part of the complex process of hypertension control in populations. As shown in Fig. 1, the five approaches have multiple links and interactions.

The protocol prescribed only a minimum of items; participants were asked to adhere to the minimum, but to expand the information base at their discretion, with locally suitable items, whenever desirable. The protocol has been slightly revised since the project began. The original version is included in Annex 1.

The study is a promotional demonstration project. The results of the project are expected to raise more general interest in the assessment of the level and quality of hypertension control in the community. The explicit purpose of the exercise is to identify the weak spots in the community control of hypertension in various countries and thus to help reinforce the process. An implicit expectation is that the concept and methods described in this project will stimulate health policy-makers routinely to introduce periodic assessment of various facets of hypertension control in the population.

References

1. Vuori, H.V. *Quality assurance of health services.* Copenhagen, WHO Regional Office for Europe, 1982 (Public Health in Europe, No. 16).
2. 1989 guidelines for the management of mild hypertension: memorandum from a WHO/ISH meeting. *Bulletin of the World Health Organization*, **67**: 493 – 498 (1989).

3

REVIEW, ANALYSIS AND COMPARISON OF SURVEY RESULTS

L. Wilhelmsen & T. Strasser

The objective of the Hypertension Management Audit Project was to analyse the current status of hypertension control in various European countries. The information obtained from the participating centres will be summarized in comparative tables. A synopsis should be both useful and necessary to establish a coherent pattern of hypertension control in selected parts of Europe.

The participating centres were free to choose from the protocol the approaches they felt were most practicable in their environment and circumstances. Table 1 summarizes which surveys were carried out where. The survey in Vernier, Switzerland (described in Chapter 12) was actually carried out as an exercise by postgraduate students of community medicine and epidemiology. It does not conform to the protocol used in the other surveys and will not therefore be included further in this comparative review.

Two reports (from Germany and India) were received too late to include in the overview. They appear as Annexes 2 and 3.

Seven countries in the European Region of WHO were involved (including Israel, a Member State of the Region since 1985). Three countries in western Europe had liberal health care systems, three others in the eastern part of Europe had completely socialized health care, while Israel stood between socialized and liberal health care. While the project was by no means intended to analyse the advantages and disadvantages of liberal versus socialized health care systems, the pattern of participation in the subprojects shows that, as may be expected, drug utilization studies are more readily carried out in countries with a centralized economy.

The characteristics of the populations in the community surveys are presented in Table 2. The surveyed population groups exceeded 150 000 individuals (excluding the large Munich population), and the random samples examined included just over 39 000 men and women. Participation rates ranged from 69% to 100%. The latter figure applies to two industrial groups in Romania, which were in effect "captive" populations. In the industrial populations there were more men than women; in random samples of the general populations there were, as may be expected, slightly more women than men. In conclusion, a large sample was surveyed with good participation rates; random samples of the general populations are representative,

Table 1. Which surveys were carried out where

Site	Chapter	Community survey	Patient survey	Consumer inquiry	Physician inquiry	Drug utilization study
Five populations in Hungary	5	+	–	+	+[a]	–
Šiška, Ljubljana, Slovenia	6	+	+	+	+[b]	–
Vicenza, Italy	7	+	+	+	+	–
Slatina and Sibiu, Romania	8	+	+	+	+	–
Siano, Italy	9	+	+	+	+	–
Ashkelon, Israel	10	+	+	+	+	–
Munich, Germany	11	+	–	–	–	–
Vernier, Switzerland	12	+	–	–	–	–
Bochum/Dortmund, Stuttgart and Munich, Germany	13	–	–	–	+	–
Stuttgart, Germany	14	–	–	–	+	–
Catalonia, Spain	15	–	–	–	+	–
Hungary	16	–	–	–	–	+
Novi Sad district, Yugoslavia (Serbia & Montenegro)	17	–	–	–	–	+
Slovenia	18	–	–	–	–	+

[a] Carried out on a national sample.

[b] Carried out in Slovenia as a whole.

Table 2. Community surveys: types of population and numbers examined

Site (age range in years of study population)	Type of population	Study population		Random sample screened (aged 35 – 64)		Participation rate
		Male	Female	Male	Female	(%)
Five populations in Hungary (18+)	Random sample and industrial	39 720	36 825	8 378	6 838	88
Šiška, Ljubljana, Slovenia (35 – 69)	Random sample	18 506	21 659	1 260	1 705	84
Vicenza, Italy (35 – 64)	Random sample	5 150	5 998	1 289	1 565	70
Slatina, Romania (35 – 64)	Industrial	7 851	2 734	5 004	1 932	100
Sibiu, Romania (35 – 64)	Industrial	4 007	2 742	1 613	1 225	100
Siano, Italy (18 – 82)	Random sample	2 840	3 505	1 462	1 727	83
Ashkelon, Israel (35 – 64)	Industrial	11 000		3 012		86
Munich, Germany (30 – 69)	Random sample	524 328		1 042[a]	1 174[a]	69

[a] Aged 30 – 69.

while the industrial populations, though not representative of the background populations, are considered typical in their own settings.

Epidemiological information derived from the community surveys is presented in Table 3. The prevalence of confirmed hypertension varies widely; it is considerably lower in the industrial populations, probably due to a selection bias during recruitment for employment (known as the healthy worker effect). In the general populations (mostly aged 35 to 64 years), prevalence rates around 20% are plausible in the light of many earlier epidemiological surveys. The prevalence of 27% in the population of Vicenza is higher than expected, however, and calls for further investigation. The low rate of 5.4% in the Hungarian populations is probably due to the way the survey was carried out: only those suspected of hypertension were recalled for further examinations, as laid down in the protocol. In the other surveys, the whole sample was re-examined. Three of the Hungarian populations were also industrial groups.

A summary of the treatment status of confirmed hypertensives is presented in Table 4. The proportion of newly discovered (i.e. previously undiagnosed) hypertension varies from 10% to 34% of confirmed hypertension. This proportion is lower than the 50% of undiagnosed hypertensives generally found at the

Table 3. Community surveys: prevalence of confirmed hypertension (blood pressure > 160/95 mmHg)

Site	Total examined	Confirmed hypertension	Prevalence (%)
Five populations in Hungary	15 216	829	5.4
Šiška, Ljubljana, Slovenia	2 965	619	20.8
Vicenza, Italy	2 854	772	27.0
Slatina and Sibiu, Romania	9 774	606	6.2
Siano, Italy	3 189	765	24.0
Ashkelon, Israel	3 012	212	7.0
Munich, Germany	2 216	454	20.5

beginning of the 1970s (the rule of the halves) *(1)*, thus showing an improvement in the detection of hypertension. The proportion of previously known but untreated hypertensives varies from 22% to 38%, with the exception of the special (captive) industrial population in Romania, where all hypertensives were reported to be under treatment. Again, this proportion is a sign of a certain improvement in health care, though it is still far from optimal. If, however, the question of the adequacy of treatment is considered, the situation does not seem to have changed much since the 1970s. On average only 29% of all confirmed hypertensives have attained normal blood pressure levels. Even by adding up normotensives and borderline hypertensives as a (more liberal) criterion of adequate treatment, an average 46% of confirmed hypertensives are still being treated inadequately – much as they were some 20 years ago. The population samples from Ashkelon and Munich have been omitted from this analysis; the existence of a hypertensive detection and follow-up programme in Ashkelon makes the comparison of results invalid, while the data from Munich are not detailed enough.

Figures on overtreatment, in the few centres where they are available, should be accepted critically. This information, though highly desirable, is difficult to obtain; most centres did not use the method for obtaining it prescribed by the protocol.

Table 5 compares drug usage as revealed by the patient surveys. The pattern does not show major differences from centre to centre. Diuretics are the leading drug family, followed by beta-blockers. Rauwolfia is given in up to 9% of patients, generally in combination with other drugs. Calcium antagonists are given in 3 – 15% of patients. In the Italian centres, the recently introduced ACE inhibitors are being used in a surprisingly high proportion, showing how drug prescribing habits may change in some environments and remain more

Table 4. Community and patient surveys: treatment status of confirmed hypertensives

Site	Confirmed hypertensives (No.)	Confirmed hypertensives who are: newly discovered (%)	previously known: treated by drugs (%)	previously known: not treated (%)	Treated hypertensives whose blood pressure is: hyper-tensive (%)	border-line (%)	normo-tensive (%)	Over-treatment (%)
Five populations in Hungary	829	10	60	30	42	33	25	Not assessed
Šiška, Ljubljana, Slovenia	619	18	40[a]	38	54	29	17	7
Vicenza, Italy	772	21	51	28	48	33	19	Not assessed
Slatina, Romania	315	20	80	0	49	8	43	5 (Slatina and Sibiu combined)
Sibiu, Romania	291	17	83	0	38	14	48	
Siano, Italy	765	34	44	22	47	33	20	Not assessed

[a] Information missing in 4% (26 individuals).

conservative in others (such as the persisting use of rauwolfia).

The reports from the centres show that prescribing habits are more consistent within countries. Intercountry differences in drug prescribing are well known from the literature *(2)*.

It should be stressed that the data in Table 5, obtained from the patient survey, should be considered in conjunction with the information obtained from the physician inquiry and, in Hungary, Novi Sad and Slovenia, with the much more elaborate and solid information obtained from the drug utilization studies.

What kind of work-up for hypertensive patients is used in various countries? Table 6 compares four centres in this respect, and reveals considerable intercentre differences. The proportion of patients subjected to body weight measurements ranges from 35% to 96%, chest X-rays from 43% to 92%, eyeground examinations from 11% to 70%, serum cholesterol measurements from 27% to 92%, and serum potassium measurements from 0% to 59%. While chest X-rays are performed in 43 – 92%, information on alcohol intake is requested at the most in 58% of patients and in some cases not at all. Yet X-raying is expensive and potentially harmful, and contributes very little to diagnosis or treatment. Alcohol, on the other hand, is a contributing factor to hypertension and hypertensive patients should not drink.

Table 5. Patient surveys: proportions of patients given various antihypertensive drugs[a]

Drug group	Percentage of patients in:				
	Slatina	Sibiu	Šiška	Vicenza	Siano
Beta-blockers	29	28	20	16	15
Diuretics	34	29	24	41	45
Vasodilators	8	13	10	11	–
Rauwolfia	9	3	6	–	5
Calcium antagonists	9	5	7	3	15
Centrally acting sympathicolytics	5	3	17	11	5
Others	6[b]	19[b]	17	18[b]	15[c]

[a] Combination therapy adjusted so figures do not exceed 100%.
[b] Mainly ACE inhibitors.
[c] All ACE inhibitors.

A clear doctrine is obviously needed in the matter of the diagnosis and management of hypertension. The recommendations of WHO and ISH *(3)* do not seem to have had a visible impact in this domain.

Table 7 is an attempt to summarize the results of the consumer inquiry. The questionnaire on which this information is based was elaborated several years ago, before the recent developments in the methodology of assessing quality of life, and will be revised if the project continues. Nevertheless, despite being simplistic, these questions give some insight into the patients' self-perceptions and some of their perceptions of the health care they are receiving. Considerable differences seem to exist between centres in this respect, but they are not necessarily related to health care *per se*, and could be due to cultural differences between various countries and societies.

The physician inquiry has met with the greatest acceptance among the five approaches of the project. As seen in Table 8, eight inquiries were conducted with a total of 2465 physicians out of a sample of 4830, drawn from a total number of 8281 physicians. In Stuttgart, two separate physician inquiries were carried out on basically the same sample: one by U. Keil and his collaborators comparing Stuttgart with Bochum/Dortmund and Munich (Chapter 13) and the other by A. Füller and his collaborators looking at discrepancies between attitudes and self-reported behaviour in Stuttgart alone (Chapter 14).

Table 6. Patient surveys: proportion of patients with previously diagnosed hypertension subjected to various procedures

Procedure	Percentage of patients in:			
	Slatina and Sibiu	Šiška	Vicenza	Siano
Clinical work-up				
Body weight	96	54	49	35
Height	96	49	47	18
Urine analysis	98	81	63	62
Electrocardiogram	98	81	59	54
Serum potassium	–	–	59	32
Serum creatinine	75	48	60	30
Serum cholesterol	92	62	63	27
Serum uric acid	30	46	59	32
Blood sugar	–	70	64	65
Oral glucose tolerance test	6	70	26	37
Chest X-ray	92	76	43	55
Eye-ground examination	70	54	29	11
Inquiry about risk factors				
Family history	94	50	61	61
Smoking habits	33	–	61	75
Alcohol consumption	35	–	58	38
Oral contraceptives use	–	–	26	14
Detection of overweight patients				
Patients overweight	18	56	47	62
Overweight patients recognized as such by physician	90	70	78	70
Advice about non-drug measures				
Weight reduction	16	39	27	20
Sodium restriction	57	48	39	30
Physical exercise	18	38	43	10
Non-drug treatment (one or more of the above)	57	80	74	52

Table 7. Consumer inquiries: summary of the results

Questions	Answers	Percentage of patients in: Five populations in Hungary	Slatina	Sibiu	Šiška	Vicenza	Siano
Is it difficult to be a patient with high blood pressure?	No	79	10	22	55	61	50
	Yes	14	72	50	33	37	40
	Hard to say	7	18	28	12	2	10
How satisfied are you with the care given previously for your high blood pressure?	Very satisfied	18	31	49	11	12	8
	Satisfied	70	54	49	63	69	18
	Not satisfied	4	10	0	20	10	38
	Very dissatisfied	1	0	0	1	5	21
	No opinion	7	5	2	5	4	15
When was the last time you took drugs for high blood pressure?	Today or yesterday	79	29	72	78	92	89
	2 – 3 days ago	10	15	4	6	5	7
	One week ago	2	18	3	3	1	3
	One week to one month ago	3	13	4	3	2	1
	More than one month ago	3	25	3	10	0	0
	Other, when?	3	0	14	0	0	0
Do you take your drugs for high blood pressure regularly?	No	21	42	36	28	26	30
	Yes	79	58	64	72	74	70
When visiting a clinic, is it important for you to meet the same doctor/nurse?	Absolutely	52	31	28	81	37	82
	Rather	34	33	33	13	41	15
	Not especially	11	21	17	6	11	3
	Not at all	1	15	6	0	10	0
	No opinion	2	0	16	0	1	0
Do you usually see the same doctor?	Always	45	30	54	80	85	88
	Often	47	41	39	10	12	10
	Seldom	7	26	7	2	3	2
	Never	0	3	0	0	1	0
	Do not know	1	0	0	8	0	0
Occasional deviations in drug taking are quite common. On average, how often during the last month have you missed your tablets (or some of them)	Never	38	64	42	45	78	53
	Once or twice in the last month	44	25	27	29	12	32
	Once a week	7	12	8	13	6	8
	Several times a week	9	14	15	7	3	5
	Nearly every day	2	13	8	5	1	2
Do you think that it is easy to remember to take the tablets as prescribed?	No	4	37	33	6	23	34
	Yes	96	63	67	94	77	66

Table 8. Physician inquiries: coverage

Site	Physicians in region (No.)	Physicians in sample (No.)	Response rate (%)	Question-naires available
Hungary	1900	381	43	164
Slovenia	950	950	43	413
Vicenza, Italy	248	248	54	135
Slatina and Sibiu, Romania	115	115	85	98
Siano, Italy	175	175	72	126
Bochum-Dortmund, Germany	442	442	71	314
Stuttgart, Germany	361	361	68	245
Munich, Germany	1251	1251	40	500
Stuttgart, Germany	480	480	68	244
Catalonia, Spain	2359	427	53	226

Although the absolute number of respondents is considerable, the overall response rate barely exceeded 50%. Still, in three inquiries the response rate was over 70%. It should be assumed, however, that the respondents were those physicians who were more interested in hypertension and its control; thus the replies probably give a slanted picture, better than the underlying reality. It should also be added that physicians' self-reports reflect their attitudes, not their actual behaviour. Self-image does not necessarily match reality. As pointed out in some individual reports, however, reality is unlikely to be better than the image given by the physicians; the information obtained is therefore a useful gauge.

Table 9 presents a wide scatter of practices in the techniques of measuring blood pressure. The use of aneroid sphygmomanometers is still widespread, and the use of automatic machines seems to be spreading but slowly.

Surprisingly, many physicians report using Korotkoff IV sounds; most round off readings at 5 mmHg (0.667 kPa), while 3 – 26% admit rounding up at 10 mmHg (1.33 kPa). About two thirds consider self-measurement by patients useful, and 40 – 97% affirm that they are teaching patients how to do this. With some empirical knowledge of the practices in various countries, this figure is probably an overstatement.

Table 10 shows an interesting variation in the majority opinion about the systolic and diastolic

Table 9. Physician inquiries: reported practices in blood pressure measurement

Reported practices	Percentage of physicians in:								
	Hungary	Slatina and Sibiu	Slovenia	Catalonia	Bochum/ Dortmund	Stuttgart	Munich	Vicenza	Siano
Nurses measure blood pressure	32	16	27[a]	17	35[a]	26[a]	33[a]	12	10
How is blood pressure measured?									
Right arm	–	16	19	23	18	20	23	17	38
Left arm	–	12	30	37	14	15	16	16	22
Both arms	92	83	25	67	22	20	22	44	5
Sitting	83	62	72	81	61	66	72	46	27
Lying	–	34	16	7	3	5	2	10	45
Standing	2	4	2	2	1	0	0	9	4
It varies	15	–	10	5	34	29	24	34	–
At least 5 minutes' interval between blood pressure measurements	62	40	–	–	–	–	–	51	31
Blood pressure measuring device									
Mercury sphygmomanometer	42	43	87	68	–	–	–	81	75
Automatic	3	0	1	0	–	–	–	–	2
Aneroid sphygmomanometer	5	57	12	31	–	–	–	9	23
How often is instrument standardized?									
Once a year	40	90	73	14	–	–	–	36	22
Once in 2 years	44	4	19	10	–	–	–	21	72
Less frequently	–	6	8	–	–	–	–	36	2
Never	16	–	–	65	–	–	–	–	4
Differential cuff sizes used	31	–	7	–	21	20	14	5	–
Diastolic reading based on:									
Korotkoff IV	21	35	22	16	37	34	34	47	18
Korotkoff V	79	59	78	78	63	66	66	38	82

Table 9 (contd)

Reported practices	Percentage of physicians in:								
	Hungary	Slatina and Sibiu	Slovenia	Catalonia	Bochum/ Dortmund	Stuttgart	Munich	Vicenza	Siano
Are values recorded to the next:									
10 mmHg	12	6	3	26	–	–	–	4	14
5 mmHg	82	34	48	70	–	–	–	70	80
2 mmHg	5	55	32	4	–	–	–	24	6
Other	1	5	17	–	–	–	–	2	–
Physician thinks self-measurement is useful	70	71	–	–	71	70	75	85	60
Physician teaches self-measurement to patients	97	59	–	–	–	–	–	81	40
Physician checked own blood pressure during past year	–	–	74	–	–	–	–	65	68

[a] Generally or often.

values that are considered indicators for starting drug treatment. While in all centres most physicians declare that they start drug treatment at 160 mmHg, the significant diastolic values are given as 95 – 100 mmHg. The scatter within centres is large, indicating once again the need to disseminate appropriate guidelines.

Most physicians in most centres ascribe high importance to nonpharmacological treatment and risk factor control. When cross-checked with information obtained from the patient survey, however (Table 6), these statements seem closer to lip-service than to reality.

Table 11 shows the physicians' replies to questions on the diagnostic and therapeutic procedures they use. The most frequent choice of drugs is as expected. In those centres where both the patient and the physician survey has been completed, however, it is interesting to compare physicians' opinions on diagnostic work-up and the reality as reflected by patient records. In general, physicians report the need for certain diagnostic methods much more often than can in fact be found in the patient records (Table 12). Naturally, since two different categories are being juxtaposed they are not strictly comparable. Nevertheless, Table 12 illustrates once again the divergence between opinions (or intentions) and actual behaviour. Since opinions reflect knowledge, it may be concluded that for physicians to be informed, although a prerequisite, does not suffice. Additional methods are needed to influence physicians' compliance; perhaps feedback from the

Table 10. Physician inquiries: reported behaviour and attitudes

Behaviour and attitudes	Hungary	Slatina and Sibiu	Slovenia	Catalonia	Vicenza	Siano
Number of patients seen per year	2000	3900	–	35[a]	700	560
Number of hypertensive patients in the practice	210	280	–	6[a]	110	89
Percentage of physicians who:						
keep a register of hypertensive patients	92	93	–	31	34	–
have a reminder system	99	92	–	–	81	–
actively invite patients for follow-up	83	98	–	–	–	–
deem a personal computer useful	70	66	–	–	61	–
Systolic blood pressure level (mmHg) considered by majority as hypertension in people aged:						
< 35 years	120	150	–	–	–	140
35 – 59 years	150/160[b]	160	–	150	–	150
60 + years	170	160	–	–	–	160
Diastolic blood pressure level (mmHg) considered by majority as hypertension in people aged:						
< 35 years	99	90	–	–	90	90
35 – 59 years	95	95	–	90	95	90
60 + years	95	95	–	–	95	90
Systolic blood pressure level (mmHg) at which majority consider drug treatment essential for people aged:						
< 35 years	–	140	–	–	–	150
35 – 59 years	–	160	160	160	–	160
60 + years	–	180	–	–	–	180
Diastolic blood pressure level (mmHg) at which majority consider treatment essential for people aged:						
< 35 years	–	95	–	–	95	95
35 – 59 years	–	100	95	100	95	95
60 + years	–	–	–	–	100	100
Percentage of physicians who advise non-drug treatment:	–	97	–	–	97	88
weight reduction	94	99	99	93	99	80
sodium restriction	90	100	97	98	95	82
physical exercise	69	78	85	63	90	61
behavioural therapy	84	98	47	–	56	–
stopping oral contraception	75	58	–	–	58	78
alcohol restriction	–	–	67	67	–	–

Table 10 (contd)

Behaviour and attitudes	Hungary	Slatina and Sibiu	Slovenia	Catalonia	Vicenza	Siano
Percentage of physicians who assess cardiovascular disease risk factors:						
smoking	99	99	–	–	99	97
hyperlipidaemia	85	97	–	–	94	99
alcohol consumption	96	94	–	–	93	93
diabetes	96	–	–	–	–	90
hyperuricaemia	57	–	–	–	–	37

[a] Number of patients per day.

[b] Both equally frequent.

present audit project and similar assessments could be used to improve performance in health care.

How do physicians obtain information on advances in the management of hypertension? Considerable differences seem to exist between various environments. According to Table 13, medical journals are the most important source of information for physicians (78 – 97% of physicians). It would definitely be of interest to check the validity of this information with more targeted inquiries. On the other hand, the importance of continuing education ranges from 20% to 90%; textbooks range from 18% to 95%, national programmes from 4% to 78%. WHO has a low profile with 13 – 24%, in only three out of nine centres. On the other hand, pharmaceutical industry information figures are high in most centres, with 58 – 92%.

A comparative analysis of the results yields interesting findings that may – and should – be used to improve policies for the control of hypertension, notwithstanding the need for further assessments in this domain.

References

1. Cardiovascular diseases: care and prevention. *WHO chronicle*, **28**: 116 – 125 (1974).
2. WHO Drug Utilization Research Group (DURG). Therapeutic traditions in Northern Ireland, Norway and Sweden: II. Hypertension. *European journal of clinical pharmacology*, **30**: 521 – 525 (1986).
3. 1989 guidelines for the management of mild hypertension: memorandum from a WHO/ISH meeting. *Bulletin of the World Health Organization*, **67**: 493 – 498 (1989).

Table 11. Physician inquiries: diagnostic and therapeutic procedures reportedly used

Procedure	Percentage of physicians in:								
	Hungary	Slatina and Sibiu[a]	Slovenia[b]	Catalonia	Bochum/ Dortmund	Stuttgart	Munich	Vicenza	Siano
Diagnostic									
Percentage of physicians who measure:									
body weight	87	85	–	67	–	–	–	93	80
height	48	57	–	38	–	–	–	51	40
urine analysis	97	90	87	66	86	92	85	95	83
electrocardiogram	90	97	83	60	84	69	80	94	92
serum potassium	61	50	50	49	57	61	52	96	43
serum creatinine	70	80	77	80	87	87	84	96	51
serum cholesterol	87	97	76	85	74	71	68	96	90
serum uric acid	52	56	62	69	55	45	54	90	51
blood sugar	85	–	79	81	58	50	58	–	80
post-load blood sugar	19	61	–	–	–	–	–	33	32
chest X-ray	41	88	59	40	48	39	43	79	68
eye-ground examination	92	98	67	60	53	51	55	86	32
Therapeutic									
Most frequent choice of monotherapy for people aged:									
< 35 years	Beta-blockers	Beta-blockers	Beta-blockers[c]	Diuretics[d]	Beta-blockers	Beta-blockers	Beta-blockers	Beta-blockers	Beta-blockers
35 – 59 years	Vaso-dilators	Diuretics	Beta-blockers[c]	Diuretics[d]	–	–	–	Equal use of all drugs	Diuretics
60 + years	Vaso-dilators	Diuretics	Diuretics	Diuretics[d]	Diuretics	Diuretics	Diuretics	Equal use of diuretics, ACE inhibitors and calcium antagonists	ACE inhibitors and calcium antagonists
Percentage of physicians who reduce dosage when blood pressure is normalized	69	93	–	–	92	92	94	53	82

[a] Not quoted in country report.

[b] Physicians were asked which procedures they considered essential for the diagnosis of hypertension.

[c] These age groups were taken together under the heading "younger patients".

[d] All age groups from 25 to 60 years.

Table 12. Physician and patient inquiries: percentage likelihood of diagnostic procedures being carried out, according to physicians' opinions and findings in patient records

Procedure	Slovenia		Slatina and Sibiu		Vicenza		Siano	
	Opinions	Records	Opinions	Records[a]	Opinions	Records	Opinions	Records
Body weight	–	54	85	96	93	49	80	35
Height	–	49	57	96	51	47	40	18
Urine analysis	87	81	90	98	95	63	83	62
Electrocardiogram	83	81	97	98	94	59	92	54
Serum potassium	50	–	50	–	96	59	43	32
Serum creatinine	77	48	80	75	96	60	51	30
Serum cholesterol	76	62	97	92	96	63	90	27
Serum uric acid	62	46	56	30	90	59	51	32
Chest X-ray	59	76	88	92	79	43	68	55
Eye-ground examination	67	54	98	70	86	29	32	11

[a] Industrial population undergoing periodic health examinations regardless of hypertension: explains the near to 100% findings.

Table 13. Physician inquiries: opinions and information

Statement	Percentage of physicians who agree in:				
	Hungary	Slatina and Sibiu	Slovenia	Vicenza	Siano
Media coverage of hypertension is adequate	38	57	...	47	...
Media supports physicians' treatment of hypertension	88	78	...	73	...
Side effects should be tolerated by patient	...	67	...	59	...
Usual sources of information					
medical journals	97	95	78	84	90
continuing education	90	37	71	64	20
textbooks	68	95	23	60	18
pharmaceutical industry	76	82	74	58	92
television/radio/newspapers	13	37	–	3	32
antihypertension leagues	–	33	–	1	...
WHO	22	24	–	13	–
ISH	–	–	–	...	–
national programmes	78	44	–	4	21
congresses	–	–	–	...	–

Note. ... = question not asked.
– = answer not given.

4

DISCUSSION

T. Strasser & L. Wilhelmsen

The control of hypertension in populations consists of a complicated series of complex operations. This complexity leads to a certain opacity, making it difficult both in practice and conceptually to assess the levels, quality, impact (effectiveness) and efficiency – and hence also the benefits and cost/benefits – of hypertension control.

There are two complementary ways of evaluating health interventions: outcome evaluation and process evaluation. Measurements are based on indicators and indices. The term "indicator" is best used for measures of simpler phenomena, and "index" for more complex ones *(1,2)*. According to this terminology, mortality due to hypertension or, for that matter, the incidence of (or mortality from) stroke, myocardial infarction and other complications of hypertension can be considered as indices of the impact or outcome of hypertension control. Hypertension is obviously only one of the factors involved, however, and therefore any one of the outcome indices is an unsatisfactory index of the impact of hypertension control. For instance, stroke mortality started declining in the United States long before the discovery of antihypertensive agents *(3)*. These indices should be used as ingredients of complex analyses, such as that to be produced by the WHO MONICA project *(4)*.

For practical purposes, for the quality assurance of health interventions *(5)*, process evaluation seems more appropriate. This is the approach taken in the present project. This type of evaluation gives access to a great number of relevant indicators, such as the proportion of awareness in the population, the percentage of missed appointments, the distribution of therapeutic attitudes among physicians, or the structure of drug prescribing, to take only a few examples. All of these measure one single detail of hypertension control but, when taken together, they produce a complex pattern, in keeping with the complexity of hypertension control itself.

Some comments on terminology should be made at this point. According to Vuori *(5)*, the term medical audit should be reserved for the retrospective assessment of the quality of care on the basis of medical records. While this term fully applies to the patient approach described in the protocol (Annex 1), assessment of the other aspects described (awareness, physicians' attitudes, patient perceptions, drug prescribing) is a way of auditing the other facets of the management of health interventions aimed at controlling hypertension in populations.

Although terminology matters, it should not be overestimated. By the same token, it does not matter to which of the four types of evaluation *(6)* the project belongs. What really matters is medical accountability *(7)*. So too does making use of the information obtained by auditing as positive feedback to correct and improve the intervention. Quality assessment should not be considered a threat, but should become an integral part of endeavours to improve care *(8)*. The information obtained by evaluation research should ultimately be used to translate the findings into health policy *(9)*, a difficult but essential task.

Patterns of Hypertension Control in Populations

The disproportion between the wealth of literature on methods of treating hypertension, especially the opportunities offered by drug therapy, and the relative paucity of evaluation research in this field is remarkable.

What is really going on in hypertension control on the international scene? The present study highlights certain points, on a pilot basis, in selected centres and environments. The information obtained needs to be put into the context of the existing literature.

The approximately 20% prevalence of hypertension, as defined in the present study, corresponds in general to that found in earlier *(10)* and more recent *(11)* WHO studies. It is lower than the figures obtained when the results of numerous epidemiological studies in Europe in the 1970s were pooled *(12)*. On the other hand, the pooled blood pressure values in the latter study were mostly the means of two measurements on a single occasion.

Of crucial importance is the level of awareness of and treatment for hypertension in populations. In the early 1970s, awareness ranged from 35% to 80% in various European countries studied by WHO, and treatment rates varied from 10% to 60% *(10)*. By the mid 1980s, treatment rates in various European centres ranged from 18% to 50% (with an average of 34%) in men and from 27% to 88% (with an average of 56%) in women *(11)*. As so often, both awareness and treatment rates were higher in women than in men. Despite the wide range, these proportions match the present audit findings rather well. Although, as pointed out in the previous chapter, the awareness rates have improved since the early 1970s, the situation is still far from satisfactory.

An analysis of the Scottish Heart Health study *(13)* shows results close to the present audit findings. The situation has been reported as unsatisfactory in the elderly population in Italy *(14)* and, despite improvements in the control of hypertension in the United States *(15)*, the problem of poor blood pressure control persists, as a "gap between the achieved and the achievable" *(16)*. To stimulate further improvements, continuing audits seem to be necessary at various levels. These can include general practices, such as the example given by two general practitioners in Wales *(17)*.

Physicians, Drugs and Patients

Disease control is the result of a vast array of factors: scientific research, cultural settings, economic development or resources, societal structures, political forces, health care, communication within societies, to mention only the most obvious ones. All these interact and influence the three elements the project is dealing with: physicians' knowledge and attitudes, the use of antihypertensive drugs and the patient.

Physicians' knowledge and attitudes have been investigated repeatedly. Besides publications by participants in the present project, based on the same set of data *(18,19)*, publications have appeared on this topic in the United States and some European countries. A survey of 2960 physicians in the United States (based on a sample of 100 000 general practitioners and internists) reported on their knowledge of correlates of hypertension, methods of diagnosing hypertension, and therapeutic habits. These findings showed a satisfactory level of (self-reported) behaviour *(20)*. A more recent survey of primary care physicians in the State of Georgia, in the United States, revealed rather energetic habits of drug usage, which correlated with the perceived influence of pharmaceutical sources of information ("drug visitors") *(21)*.

The weekly journal *Medical tribune* recently published the summary report of an inquiry into the opinions of 1350 physicians on the management of hypertension, derived from a postal inquiry. Respondents were mostly general practitioners, from ten European countries. The attitudes of the respondents differed considerably with regard to starting medication, referral criteria, diagnostic procedures and treatment of associated risk factors *(22)*. In another inquiry, members of the British Hypertension Society were sent a questionnaire asking for their views on the management of hypertensive patients. The response rate was 60%. This highly selected group of physicians was virtually in complete agreement that weight loss and alcohol restriction are effective in lowering blood pressure, but varied widely on the minimum level of blood pressure it considered warranted drug treatment *(23)*. Nevertheless, in an audit of the records of British general practitioners, weight (and smoking) control and follow-up were documented "unimpressively" *(24)*, showing once again the gap between opinions and practice.

Drug usage is the second major element in the therapeutic process. According to the British Hypertension Society study *(22)*, beta-blockers were the drugs of first choice in middle-aged patients, followed by thiazide diuretics. As described in Chapter 3, these opinions tally roughly with the findings in the various centres participating in the present project only as far as younger patients are concerned. For middle-aged patients, diuretics are the typical drug of choice. This is also documented by the drug utilization studies (Chapters 16 – 18), showing that the consumption of diuretics takes first place among the single drugs. Similar findings regarding first-choice drugs were reported, in 1982, from the United States *(25)*. In Nordic countries, on the other hand, beta-blockers precede diuretics in middle-aged patients *(26)*, and a closer look at drug usage discloses substantial differences in the proportions of the drugs chosen from other families.

Patient satisfaction is obviously a central element in the therapeutic process. It depends more on the quality of the physician's interpersonal skills than on the quantity of teaching and instruction to which patients are exposed *(27)*. More personalized care has been understood to result in better blood pressure reduction, than the rather impersonal care patients usually receive *(28)*. Interestingly, the literature on the role of patient satisfaction in the therapy of hypertension is scarce. The varied results of the present project, reviewed in the previous chapter, indicate that much more attention should be paid to this component of hypertension management. Methods of interactive communication with patients need to be fostered. These methods are the basis of patient education and physicians need more formal training in this domain *(29)*. WHO and ISH are at present proposing a project for the advancement of patient education in hypertension, on the "teaching the teacher principle" *(30)*.

References

1. Noack, H. & Abelin, T. Conceptual and methodological aspects of measurement in health and health promotion. *In*: Abelin, T. et al., ed. *Measurement in health promotion and protection*. Copenhagen, WHO Regional Office for Europe, 1987 (WHO Regional Publications, European Series, No. 22).
2. Goldberg, M. & Dab, W. Complex indexes for measuring a complex phenomenon. *In*: Abelin, T. et al., ed. *Measurement in health promotion and protection*. Copenhagen, WHO Regional Office for Europe, 1987 (WHO Regional Publications, European Series, No. 22).
3. Moriyama, I.M. et al. *Cardiovascular diseases in the United States*. Cambridge, MA, Harvard University Press, 1971.
4. WHO MONICA Project Principal Investigators. The World Health Organization MONICA project: a major international collaboration. *Journal of clinical epidemiology*, **41**: 105 – 114 (1988).
5. Vuori, H.V. *Quality assurance of health services*. Copenhagen, WHO Regional Office for Europe, 1982 (Public Health in Europe, No. 16).
6. Abramson, J.H. The four basic types of evaluation: clinical reviews and program trials. *Public health reports*, **94**: 210 – 215 (1979).
7. Gebert, A.J. Evaluation als Zwischenstufe zur Qualitätskontrolle. *In*: Gutzwiller, F. & Kocher, G., ed. *Die Qualität medizinischer Leistungen*. Zürich, SGGP, 1982 (Schriftenreihe der SGGP, No. 5).
8. Gutzwiller, F. Qualitätssicherung ärztlicher Leistungen: Definitionen und Methoden. *In*: Gutzwiller, F. & Kocher, G., ed. *Die Qualität medizinischer Leistungen*. Zürich, SGGP, 1982 (Schriftenreihe der SGGP, No. 5).
9. Sechrest, L. & Mabe, P.E. Translating evaluation research findings into health policy. *Health policy quarterly*, **1**: 57 – 72 (1981).
10. *Report of the meeting of investigators on community control of arterial hypertension, Geneva, 1 – 3 December 1980*. Geneva, World Health Organization, 1980 (unpublished document CVD/88.3).
11. WHO MONICA Project. Geographical variation in the major risk factors of coronary heart disease in men and women aged 35 – 64 years. *World health statistics quarterly*, **41**: 115 – 140 (1988).
12. ERICA Research Group. The CHD risk-map of Europe. The lst report of the WHO-ERICA Project. *European heart journal*, **9**(Suppl. 1) (1988).
13. Smith, W.C.S. et al. Control of blood pressure in Scotland: the rule of the halves. *British medical journal*, **300**: 981 – 983 (1990).
14. Avanzini, F. et al. Awareness, treatment and control of hypertension in the elderly in a general practice experience. *Clinical cardiology*, **12**: 283 – 288 (1989).
15. Subcommittee on Definition and Prevalence of the Joint National Committee on Detection, Evaluation and Treatment of High Blood Pressure. Hypertension prevalence and the status of awareness, treatment, and control in the United States. *Hypertension*, **11**(2): 209A – 222A (1988).
16. Winickoff, R.N. & Murphy, P.K. The persistent problem of poor blood pressure control. *Archives of internal medicine*, **147**: 1393 – 1396 (1987).
17. Taffinder, A.P. & Taffinder, G.A. An audit of hypertension in general practice. *Practitioner*, **228**: 595 – 598 (1984).

18. Härtel, U. et al. Hypertoniediagnose und Hypertonietherapie in der Praxis von niedergelassenen Ärzten. *Deutsches Ärzteblatt*, **84**: 632 – 641 (1987).
19. Weiland, S.K. et al. Diagnosis and management of hypertension by physicians in the Federal Republic of Germany. *Journal of hypertension*, **9**: 131 – 134 (1991).
20. Public Health Service, National Institutes of Health. *Diagnosis and management of hypertension. A nationwide survey of physicians' knowledge, attitudes, and reported behaviours*. Washington, DC, US Department of Health, Education, and Welfare, 1979 (DHEW Publication No. (NIH)79-1056).
21. McClellan, W. et al. Correlates of drug therapy of diastolic blood pressure between 80 – 89 mmHg by physicians in the community. *American journal of hypertension*, **2**: 869 – 871 (1989).
22. Hypertonie in Europa. *Medical tribune (Schweiz)*, No. 15, 12 April 1990.
23. Waller, P.C. et al. British Hypertension Society members' views on the management of hypertension patients: results of the 1988 questionnaire. *Journal of hypertension*, **8**: 931 (1990).
24. Mant, D. et al. Three year follow up of patients with raised blood pressure identified at health checks in general practice. *British medical journal*, **298**: 1360 – 1362 (1989).
25. Grimm, R.H. et al. Long-term effects of a blood pressure survey on patient treatment in a community. *Circulation*, **65**: 946 – 950 (1982).
26. WHO Drug Utilization Research Group (DURG). Therapeutic traditions in Northern Ireland, Norway and Sweden: II Hypertension. *European journal of clinical pharmacology*, **30**: 521 – 525 (1986).
27. Bartlett, E.E. et al. The effects of physician communication skills on patient satisfaction, recall, and adherence. *Journal of chronic diseases*, **37**: 755 – 764 (1984).
28. Hovell, M.F. et al. Personalized versus usual care of previously uncontrolled hypertensive patients: an exploratory analysis. *Preventive medicine*, **15**: 673 – 678 (1986).
29. Grueninger, U.J. & Strasser, T., ed. Educating the hypertensive patient – teaching the teacher. *Journal of human hypertension*, **4**(Suppl. 1) (1990).
30. *The patient education project (PEP): a cross-cultural project for the promotion and evaluation of health care in hypertension. A joint WHO/WHL project protocol.* Geneva, World Health Organization, 1989 (unpublished document CVD/89.2).

PART 2

COUNTRY PROJECTS

5

FIVE POPULATIONS IN HUNGARY

E. Török & J. Duba

Organized and coordinated by the Hungarian Institute of Cardiology, the project in Hungary included four approaches. The community survey and the consumer inquiry were carried out in five centres throughout Hungary. The physician inquiry was done on a national sample, as was the drug utilization study (see Chapter 16).

Community Survey

The community survey took place in samples of two general populations and three industrial populations.

The Csepel Iron and Metal Works is a major industrial plant on the outskirts of the city of Budapest. About 80% of the staff are engaged in heavy physical work, many of them in the iron foundry, producing items such as components of bridges and machines. At the time of the survey, the factory had about 15 000 employees. Most workers live in the industrial settlement near the factory. They are well covered by the factory health services, with about one physician per 1000 workers. The health personnel take care of both clinical medicine and occupational health, and the general practitioners are supported by a network of specialists. When on sick leave, however, workers are referred to the general practitioner near their home.

The Beloniannisz Telecommunication Instrument Factory is another industrial plant in Budapest. With nearly 3000 employees, predominantly women, this light industry produces instruments and other equipment for telecommunications. Most employees are skilled workers and 20% work in administration.

Collaborators: L. Béleczky, Health Service of Csepel Iron and Metal Works, Budapest, Hungary; A. Gálfrik, Health Service of Beloniannisz Telecommunication Instrument Factory, Budapest, Hungary; J. Kishegyi, National Institute of Health Promotion, Budapest, Hungary; A. Kovács, Department of Internal Medicine, City Hospital, Szentes, Hungary; K. Netkovszky, Health Service of Beloniannisz Telecommunication Instrument Factory, Budapest, Hungary; J. Pásztor, Computer programmer; Z. Slezák, Health Service of Csepel Iron and Metal Works, Budapest, Hungary; I. Varga, Department of Internal Medicine, County Hospital, Miskolc, Hungary; Gy. Zeltner, Department of Internal Medicine, County Hospital, Miskolc, Hungary.

Levinváros is a chemical plant with over 4000 workers, some 200 km north-east of Budapest, that produces mainly fertilizers. Many of the workers commute from the surrounding rural settlements and thus have a strong agricultural background.

One sample from a general population was taken from a suburb of Budapest, Rákoscsaba, with nearly 50 000 inhabitants over 18 years of age. It is a residential area, comprising both one-family houses surrounded by small gardens and blocks of flats run as government housing projects. The population is a mixture of lower middle class residents and industrial workers.

The other sample of nearly 5500 adults came from two typical small agricultural villages, Felgyö and Nagymágocs, whose populations consist of farmers and their families. Their eating habits are traditional, and food is prepared at home.

The size of these five populations is given in Table 1. Samples were drawn at random from men and women aged 18 – 70 years from the populations at the Csepel Works, in the suburb of Rákoscsaba and the two villages of Felgyö and Nagymágocs (with no upper age limit in the two villages). Exhaustive samples were taken in the Beloniannisz Factory and the Leninváros chemical plant. The total study population comprised some 76 000 people; the sample invited to the survey included over 17 000 men and women. With over 15 000 people attending the first examination, an overall response rate of 88% was achieved. The sample surveyed is thus representative (Table 1).

The age composition of the total study population, the sample drawn, and the sample examined are given in Table 2. Men and women are equitably represented. The elderly population is partially truncated owing to the age limits in the occupational groups, retirement age in Hungary being 55 years for women and 60 years for men. There were no marked differences between the response rates of men and women.

Table 1. Community survey, Hungary: five study populations and samples, and response rate

Population	Study population (No.)			Sample drawn (No.)			Sample screened (No.)			Response rate (%)		
	Male	Female	Total	Male	Female	Total	Male	Female	Total	Male	Female	Total
Csepel Iron and Metal Works	9 393	5 282	14 675	2 942	1 734	4 676	2 586	1 512	4 098	88	87	88
Beloniannisz Telecommunication Instrument Factory	1 337	1 625	2 962	1 337	1 625	2 962	1 204	1 493	2 697	90	92	91
Leninváros	2 609	1 430	4 039	2 609	1 430	4 039	2 577	1 401	3 978	99	98	98
Rákoscsaba	23 767	25 717	49 484	1 895	2 033	3 928	1 338	1 525	2 863	71	75	73
Felgyö and Nagymágocs	2 614	2 771	5 385	761	976	1 737	673	907	1 580	88	93	91
Total	39 720	36 825	76 545	9 544	7 798	17 342	8 378	6 838	15 216	88	88	88

A total of 15 216 people were seen at the first screening examination. Of these, 3698 (24%) had a history of elevated blood pressure, or had elevated blood pressure at the survey, or were currently on hypotensive drug treatment (Table 3). They alone were recalled for further examination.

These 3698 people had a remarkably high rate of awareness: only 7% of the women had never been told that they had high blood pressure, while the proportion of men was twice as high as that of women (15%). This was still low in comparison with findings before the widespread introduction of hypertension control activities in the 1970s.

One might expect that such a high rate of awareness would be associated with a similarly high rate of treatment. This, however, was not the case: only 43% of those found to be hypertensive were currently under treatment, while 82% had received some treatment at some time but, obviously, half of them had discontinued. Nevertheless, as a reflection of the total population, the treatment rate was high: 7% of all men and 12% of all women in the population were on antihypertensive treatment at the time of the survey. Extrapolated to the total population of Hungary (10.5 million inhabitants), the country is presumably treating over three quarters of a million hypertensive patients.

The diagnosis of hypertension should be made only after repeated examinations. The project protocol prescribes two re-examinations, to exclude transitory blood pressure elevations in individuals found to be in the hypertensive range at the first examination. Thus the 3698 people with suspected hypertension were recalled for a second and third examination. The response rate to the recalls was, unexpectedly, only 63% (Table 4) in contrast to the rather satisfactory response to the first screening examination. People found to be hypertensive on screening thus do not seem to be particularly motivated to reappear for control examinations. On reflection, however, this phenomenon should not be unexpected since 89% of them had already at some time been told they were hypertensive. Even if the proportion of drop-outs (37%) is divided by two (i.e. by the number of visits they were invited to attend) the percentage is still higher than that of the non-responders to the first screening examination.

In consequence, the final results of the community survey refer to 2335 people, whose blood pressures were measured on at least three occasions (Table 5). The effects of the re-examinations on the categorization of the individuals originally screened as hypertensive were considerable. One third now fell into the normotensive group, one third into the borderline and one third only remained in the hypertensive group.

Only 8% of the normotensives turned out to be true negatives, in other words they had never been told that they had elevated blood pressure. Thus 92% of the normotensives were false positives; they had been told they had hypertension, though repeated examinations disproved this. Even more important, 74% of the normotensives had received antihypertensive therapy at some time, including 37% who were currently on antihypertensive treatment. Some of these may, of course, be hypertensive patients whose blood pressure had been normalized by adequate treatment.

Of the 2117 subjects told at some time that they had hypertension, 301 (14%) were never treated, 639 (30%) had been treated but not currently, and 1117 (56%) were currently on antihypertensive treatment (Table 6).

Nearly half of those ever told they were hypertensive and treated in the past (but not currently) had normal blood pressure values at re-examination; the diagnosis of hypertension was confirmed in 27%, while the rest (another 27%) were borderline. Of

Table 2. Community survey, Hungary: age and sex composition of study population and samples

Age (years)	Study population						Sample drawn					
	Male		Female		Total		Male		Female		Total	
	No.	(%)	No.	(%)	No.	(%)	No.	(%)	No.	(%)	No.	(%)
18 – 24	5 030	(13)	3 713	(10)	8 743	(11.4)	1 065	(11.2)	671	(8.6)	1 736	(10.0)
25 – 34	8 694	(22)	8 290	(22)	16 984	(22.2)	2 097	(22.0)	1 621	(20.8)	3 718	(21.4)
35 – 44	10 134	(26)	9 766	(2)	19 900	(26.0)	2 416	(25.3)	2 338	(30.0)	4 754	(27.4)
45 – 54	8 411	(21)	7 109	(19)	15 520	(20.3)	2 358	(24.7)	2 015	(25.8)	4 373	(25.2)
55 – 64	5 320	(13)	4 620	(13)	9 850	(12.9)	1 302	(13.6)	788	(10.1)	2 090	(12.1)
65 +	2 221	(6)	3 327	(9)	5 548	(7.2)	306	(3.2)	365	(4.7)	671	(3.9)
All ages (18 – 65 +)	39 720	(100)	36 825	(100)	76 545	(100)	9 544	(100)	7 798	(100)	17 342	(100)

those who had been told at some time that they had hypertension, 40% had normal blood pressure values at first screening. Among those currently being treated, relatively few (25%) had normal blood pressure values, while 42% were still in the hypertensive range. A large proportion of hypertensive patients must be receiving inadequate treatment (Table 6).

Only 10% of the hypertensives had never before been told that they had hypertension. These newly discovered hypertensive patients are false negatives.

Among the true positives – hypertensives who were aware of their condition – only 494 out of 744 (66%) were on actual treatment. Available information does not allow us to conclude whether this rate is adequate or too low, as no in-depth analysis of patient management has been carried out (see the patient survey in the protocol, Annex 1).

There were 69 newly discovered borderline patients and 85 hypertensives (Table 5). They constitute 1% of the total sample screened. It is debatable whether a 1% yield of mostly mild cases of hypertension would justify mass screening. The issue can be clarified by further inquiry into how the diagnosis of hypertension was missed in these individuals before the survey. Table 7 presents information of this kind, collected during the consumer inquiry.

Consumer Inquiry

A self-administered questionnaire was handed out to the 154 newly detected hypertensive patients. Replies were obtained from 94 patients (a 61% response rate). There seems to be no difference in type of response between patients with mild and with established hypertension; they will therefore be considered together. Only 16% had not seen a

Table 2 (contd)

Age (years)	Sample screened					
	Male		Female		Total	
	No.	(%)	No.	(%)	No.	(%)
18–24	881	(10.5)	549	(8.0)	1 430	(9.4)
25–34	1 863	(22.2)	1 396	(20.4)	3 259	(21.4)
35–44	2 145	(25.6)	2 080	(30.5)	4 225	(27.8)
45–54	2 126	(25.4)	1 849	(27.0)	3 975	(26.1)
55–64	1 121	(13.4)	649	(9.5)	1 770	(11.6)
65 +	242	(2.9)	315	(4.6)	557	(3.7)
All ages (18–65 +)	8 378	(100)	6 838	(100)	15 216	(100)

doctor in the preceding two years. Blood pressure had been measured in the preceding two years in 69%. It was found elevated but the finding probably ignored in 36%. Blood pressure was said to be normal in 26%, the value had not been communicated to the patient in 7%, and no measurement was taken in 15%.

As anticipated on the basis of the high awareness, these findings show that mass screening would help diagnose only a third of the previously undetected cases of hypertension. Calculated on the total sample size, this corresponds to a possible screening yield of 0.3% – a very modest effect indeed. At present, mass screening in the Hungarian population would not be justified.

In conclusion, hypertension care in the communities studied is characterized by a high rate of awareness. Concomitantly, the confirmed hypertensives are receiving a relatively high rate of inadequate treatment. Few, if any, of the currently treated subjects appear to be overtreated. Nevertheless, a high proportion (40%) of currently normotensive subjects said they had undergone treatment earlier, although their need for therapy was not substantiated by the survey.

Considering the high rate of awareness, mass screening does not seem to be justified in these populations.

Physician Inquiry

An inquiry into the knowledge, opinions and attitudes of physicians concerning hypertension was carried out in a national sample of practising physicians.

The Hungarian Scientific Society of General Practitioners has 1900 members, about one third of the general practitioners in the country. Out of this

Table 3. Community survey, Hungary: awareness and treatment status on first screening examination

Awareness and treatment status	Male			Female			Total		
	No.	% of sample screened	% of hyper-tensives	No.	% of sample screened	% of hyper-tensives	No.	% of sample screened	% of hyper-tensives
Total sample screened	8 378	100		6 838	100		15 216	100	
Total found hypertensive at first screening	1 785	21	100	1 913	28	100	3 698	24	100
Never told	274	3	15	140	2	7	414	3	11
Told at some time	1 511	18	85	1 773	2.6	93	3 284	22	89
Treated now or in the past	1 180	14	78	1 502	22	85	2 682	18	82
Treated now	573	7	38	849	12	48	1 422	9	43

Table 4. Community survey, Hungary: subjects lost from first and second re-examinations

	Male	Female	Total
Recalled after first screening examination	1785	1913	3698
Did not reappear to first or second recall	671	692	1363
(% lost)	(38)	(36)	(37)
Final total re-examined	1114	1221	2335

Table 5. Community survey, Hungary: awareness and treatment status by blood pressure categories after two re-examinations

Awareness and treatment status	Normotensive			Borderline			Hypertensive			Total	
	No.	% of suspected hypertensives re-examined	% of normotensives	No.	% of suspected hypertensives re-examined	% of borderlines	No.	% of suspected hypertensives re-examined	% of hypertensives	No.	% of suspected hypertensives re-examined
Total re-examined	802	34	100	704	30	100	829	36	100	2335	100
Never told	64	30	8	69	31	10	85	39	10	218	100
Told at some time	738	35	92	635	30	90	744	35	90	2117	100
Treated now or in the past	591	33	74	560	30	80	665	37	80	1816	100
Treated now	299	25	37	384	33	54	494	42	60	1177	100

Table 6. Community survey, Hungary: treatment status of people told at some time they were hypertensive, and their confirmed blood pressure category after two re-examinations

Treatment status	Normotensive			Borderline			Hypertensive			Total		
	No.	% of those told they were hypertensive	% of normotensives	No.	% of those told they were hypertensive	% of borderlines	No.	% of those told they were hypertensive	% of hypertensives	No.	% of those told they were hypertensive	% of confirmed blood pressure category
Never treated	147	49	20	75	25	12	79	26	11	301	100	14
Treated in the past	292	46	40	176	27	28	171	27	23	639	100	30
Treated now	299	25	40	384	33	60	494	42	66	1177	100	56
Total	738	35	100	635	30	100	744	35	100	2117	100	100

Table 7. Consumer inquiry, Hungary: reasons given by patients for why hypertension was not diagnosed earlier

Status	Newly detected patients					
	Borderline		Hypertensive		Total	
	No.	(%)	No.	(%)	No.	(%)
Subjects were last medically examined over 2 years ago	6	(15)	9	(16)	15	(16)
Subjects were medically examined within the last 2 years, but blood pressure was not measured	2	(5)	12	(22)	14	(15)
Blood pressure was measured within the last 2 years and was normal	12	(31)	12	(22)	24	(26)
Blood pressure was measured within the last 2 years and found to be elevated	17	(44)	17	(31)	34	(36)
Blood pressure was measured but the subject was not told its value	2	(5)	5	(9)	7	(7)
Total	39	(100)	55	(100)	94	(100)

number, 400 physicians were selected at random. They received the self-administered questionnaire described in the protocol, with slight modifications.

A total of 183 questionnaires were returned (a 45% response rate); of these, 19 were analysed separately because they were not completed by practising physicians but by medical doctors of other profiles, such as administrators or hospital-based physicians. The replies of 164 practising physicians are analysed below.

The mean age of the respondents was 49 years (SD ± 9), ranging from 30 to 74 years. There were 73% male against 27% female doctors. There were 99 specialists among the responders, with 61 specialists in general medicine, 21 in internal medicine and 17 in other fields. Thus, the opinions and attitudes described are not representative of typical general practitioners in the country, but rather reflect the thinking of physicians with above average qualifications. This is due both to the fact that the sample was taken from members of the Scientific Society of General Practitioners, and that better qualified and more interested physicians were more likely to respond.

Table 8 describes the techniques of blood pressure measurement used by the physicians. Blood pressure in hypertensive patients is measured at each visit. Blood pressure measurement is less frequent in patients seeing the doctor for other reasons. Only 3% of the respondents reported using an aneroid instrument and 6% an automatic instrument; all the others use mercury sphygmomanometers. They standardize the instruments relatively often. Most doctors round off blood pressure readings at 5 mmHg. They seem to have a healthy concern for their own blood pressure, and 13% reported having hypertension themselves.

Table 9 presents the physicians' perceptions of the criteria to be used to define hypertension. The cut-off levels are definitely age-related. In younger individuals, most physicians consider that hypertension starts with systolic blood pressure above 140 mmHg. Most physicians place the beginning of hypertension in older age around 150 – 160 over 95 – 100 mmHg. The physicians believe the diastolic criterion for hypertension increases considerably with age.

Table 10 gives information on the physicians' practices and the number of patients seen. Typically, physicians see about 200 hypertensive patients per year.

Table 11 summarizes the physicians' attitudes towards non-drug treatment. There is no way of checking how far these attitudes coincide with therapeutic action. Table 12 shows that, according to the physicians' current thinking, hypertension requires an elaborate diagnostic work-up.

The preferences of physicians for the various drug families are shown in Table 13. Beta-blockers are the most frequent choice for younger patients. Vasodilators and calcium antagonists are used more extensively in older age groups. Though no time series of observations are available, the use of diuretics seems to be regressing considerably.

Table 8. Physician inquiry, Hungary:
reported practices in blood pressure measurement

Reported practices	Percentage of physicians
Blood pressure measured:	
in hypertensive patient at each visit	97
in every new patient	85
in every patient once a year	60
Measurement taken:	
by physician	68
by nurse	32
Measurement on both arms:	
occasionally	70
regularly	23
Routine measurement:	
in sitting position	83
in various positions	15
Measurement in new patients:	
in sitting position	66
in various positions	33
Measurement in patients receiving antihypertensive drugs:	
in sitting position	52
in various positions	43
Blood pressure measured:	
only once	43
more than once	57
Interval between measurements more than 5 minutes	62
Device used	
mercury	91
aneroid	3
automatic	6
Device standardized:	
once a year	40
less often	44
never	16

Reported practices	Percentage of physicians
Cuffs used	
standard cuffs only	58
differential cuffs	31
Sounds used	
Korotkoff V	79
Korotkoff IV	21
Values rounded off:	
at 10 mmHg	12
at 5 mmHg	82
at 2 mmHg	5
Self-measurement considered useful	70
Physician's own blood pressure checked:	
less than 1 month ago	35
1 – 6 months ago	37
6 – 12 months ago	16
years ago	9
never	3
Physician has hypertension	13
Does not know	4

Table 9. Physician inquiry, Hungary: blood pressure levels physicians use to define hypertension

Blood pressure (mmHg)	Cumulative percentage of physicians who define various blood pressure levels as hypertension in patients aged:		
	< 35 years	35 – 59 years	60 + years
Systolic			
> 120	12	–	–
> 140	68	17	5
> 150	90	57	28
> 160	100	96	81
> 170	100	100	94
> 180	100	100	100
Diastolic			
> 80	9	–	–
> 85	20	3	1
> 90	65	37	20
> 95	85	74	59
> 100	100	96	94
> 105	100	98	95
> 110	100	100	100

Table 10. Physician inquiry, Hungary: information about physicians' practices

Features of the practice	Percentage of physicians
Number of inhabitants covered by practice	
1 000 – 2 000	40
2 000 – 2 500	31
2 500 – 3 000	21
over 3 000	5
Number of consultations over the past year	
less than 5 000	4
5 000 – 10 000	42
10 000 – 15 000	40
more than 15 000	10
Number of hypertensive patients seen last year	
less than 100	16
100 – 200	30
200 – 300	29
300 – 400	8
over 400	8
Keeps a register of hypertensive patients	92
Has a reminder system	99
Sends out reminders	83
Does not send out reminders	16
Physician thinks personal computer would be useful	70

Table 11. Physician inquiry, Hungary: attitudes towards non-drug therapy as reflected by actions reported by physicians

Reported action	Percentage of physicians
Advise non-drug treatment	
weight reduction	94
sodium restriction	90
physical exercise	69
behavioural therapy	84
stopping oral contraception	75
Assess cardiovascular disease risk factors	
smoking	99
hyperlipidaemia	85
alcohol consumption	96
diabetes	96
hyperuricaemia	57

Table 12. Physician inquiry, Hungary: procedures performed in the clinical work-up of hypertensive patients

Procedure	Percentage of physicians who perform this procedure: at first work-up	at each annual work-up
Body weight	87	85
Height	48	22
Urine analysis	97	94
Electrocardiogram	90	85
Serum potassium	61	59
Serum creatinine	70	57
Serum cholesterol	87	80
High density lipoprotein cholesterol	29	24
Serum uric acid	52	44
Serum triglyceride	64	55
Fasting blood sugar	85	76
Post-load blood sugar	19	15
Chest X-ray	41	35
Eye-ground examination	92	83

Table 13. Physician inquiry, Hungary: physicians' first choice of drugs

Drug	Percentage of physicians who use various drugs as a first choice in patients aged:		
	< 35 years	35 – 59 years	60 + years
Beta-blockers	57	11	7
Diuretics	9	6	8
Vasodilators	2	29	23
Calcium antagonists	2	10	16
ACE inhibitors	1	2	5
Combinations	12	20	9
Other	8	15	25
No answer	9	7	7

6

ŠIŠKA, A SUBURB OF LJUBLJANA, SLOVENIA

P. Jezeršek, R. Accetto, B. Cibič, J. Dobovišek, P. Dolenc, B. Kolšek, Z. Kralj, Z. Lapanja, M. Mihelič-Brčič, J. Petrin, O. Pirc-Čerček, L. Zaletel-Kragelj & A. Žemva

The project in Slovenia included all five approaches. The community survey, the patient survey and the consumer inquiry were carried out in Siska, a suburb of Ljubljana, while the physician inquiry was carried out in Slovenia as a whole, as was the drug utilization study (see Chapter 18).

The republic of Slovenia, with about two million inhabitants, is adjacent to Croatia in the east, and bordering on Austria and Italy to the west. Ljubljana, the capital, is an administrative and industrial centre of some 600 000 inhabitants. The urban centre has merged with its surroundings, transforming the agricultural settlements around the city into the capital's suburbs. One of these suburbs, the community of Šiška, was chosen as the site of the community survey, the patient survey and the consumer inquiry.

Community Survey

Šiška is a semi-urban, semi-rural community with 88 000 inhabitants. When the survey began, the registry of inhabitants comprised 40 165 people aged 35 – 69 years (Table 1). Of these, 3549 people were selected by computer at random for the sample to be surveyed; 2965 responded to the invitation (an 84% response rate).

The results are given in Table 2. Normotensive blood pressure was defined as levels below 140/90 mmHg; borderline was defined as 140 – 159 mmHg and/or 90 – 94 mmHg; and hypertensive as over 160/95 mmHg. The defined blood pressure was based on the mean value of all measurements taken at both re-examinations. The total sample screened was re-examined twice. After the two re-examinations, 619 people or 21% were confirmed to be in the hypertensive range, and 853 people or 29% were confirmed to be borderline. Only 50% of the sample had normal blood pressures.

Among the normotensives, 18% or 273 people had at some time been told that they had elevated blood pressure; they can be considered as having been overdiagnosed. Some 8% of the normotensives (127 people) had received antihypertensive treatment at some time; they can be considered as cases of overtreatment. Finally, 5% of the normotensives (78 people) were actually under treatment at the

Table 1. Community survey, Šiška:
age and sex composition of study population and samples, and response rate

Age (years)	Study population						Sample drawn					
	Male		Female		Total		Male		Female		Total	
	No.	(%)	No.	(%)	No.	(%)	No.	(%)	No.	(%)	No.	(%)
35 – 44	6 327	(34)	6 793	(31)	13 120	(33)	487	(30)	474	(25)	961	(27)
45 – 54	6 084	(33)	6 506	(30)	12 590	(31)	587	(36)	648	(34)	1 235	(35)
55 – 64	4 329	(23)	5 484	(25)	9 813	(24)	422	(26)	601	(32)	1 023	(29)
65 – 69	1 766	(10)	2 876	(13)	4 642	(12)	154	(9)	176	(9)	330	(9)
All ages	18 506	(100)	21 659	(100)	40 165	(100)	1 650	(100)	1 899	(100)	3 549	(100)

time of the survey; this group may include both adequately treated and overtreated individuals.

Among those found to be in the hypertensive range, 137 or 22% were unaware of their condition. Of these, 111 had never been told before that they had high blood pressure; these are cases of underdiagnosis. The rest (26 people) did not remember whether they had ever been told they had hypertension; they should be considered as inappropriately managed patients. Among those confirmed as hypertensive, 345 people (56%) had received antihypertensive treatment at some time, but only 247 (40%) were under treatment at the time of the survey. As their blood pressures were still in the hypertensive range, they may be considered as being undertreated.

The epidemiological and health care situation in the population of Šiška can thus be summed up as showing a pattern of high prevalence of hypertension, associated with relatively low awareness of the condition, and with a mixture of definitely low treatment coverage (40%) and of a non-negligible rate of overdiagnosis and overtreatment, including unnecessary drug treatment.

Patient Survey

Table 3 sums up why hypertension was not discovered earlier, based on the interpretations of both the hypertensive subjects and the interviewer (a physician or nurse). Not all the replies could be categorized, so the total number of patient and interviewer replies do not match.

The various reasons are equally distributed among borderline and established hypertensives; thus the degree of blood pressure elevation does not seem to play a role. The perceptions of the reasons, however, differ considerably. While the interviewers blame mainly the overloading of the health services, patients perceive doctors' lack of interest and their overload as equally important reasons. The interviewers blame the patients' lack of interest slightly more. Patients' anxiety or reticence about having their blood pressure measured does not

Table 1 (contd)

Age (years)	Sample screened						Response rate		
	Male		Female		Total		Male	Female	Total
	No.	(%)	No.	(%)	No.	(%)	(%)	(%)	(%)
35 – 44	196	(15)	332	(19)	528	(18)	(40)	(70)	(55)
45 – 54	557	(44)	622	(37)	1 179	(40)	(95)	(96)	(95)
55 – 64	409	(32)	591	(35)	1 000	(34)	(97)	(98)	(98)
65 – 69	98	(8)	160	(9)	258	(9)	(64)	(91)	(78)
All ages	1 260	(100)	1 705	(100)	2 965	(100)	(76)	(90)	(84)

Table 2. Community survey, Šiška: awareness and treatment status by blood pressure categories after two re-examinations

Awareness and treatment status	Normotensive			Borderline			Hypertensive			Total	
	No.	% of sample screened	% of normo-tensives	No.	% of sample screened	% of border-lines	No.	% of sample screened	% of hyper-tensives	No.	% of sample screened
Total sample screened	1493	50	100	853	29	100	619	21	100	2965	100
Never told	1133	38	76	479	16	56	111	4	18	1723	58
Not sure whether told	87	3	6	49	2	6	26	1	4	162	5
Told at some time	273	9	18	325	11	38	482	16	78	1080	36
Treated now or in the past	127	4	8	200	7	23	345	12	56	672	23
Treated now	78	3	5	133	4	16	247	8	40	458	15

Table 3. Patient survey, Šiška: reasons given by patients and interviewers for why hypertension was not diagnosed earlier

Reason	Borderline				Hypertensive				Total			
	Patient		Interviewer		Patient		Interviewer		Patient		Interviewer	
	No.	(%)	No.	(%)	No.	(%)	No.	(%)	No.	(%)	No.	(%)
Overload of health services	49	(27)	79	(43)	40	(30)	70	(46)	89	(28)	149	(45)
Physician's lack of interest when seen by patient for other reason	49	(24)	3	(2)	34	(25)	1	(1)	77	(25)	4	(1)
Patient's lack of interest	39	(22)	50	(28)	30	(22)	41	(27)	69	(22)	91	(27)
Patients do not see the doctor when feeling well	35	(20)	37	(21)	26	(19)	28	(18)	61	(20)	65	(20)
Patient's fears	12	(7)	11	(6)	5	(4)	12	(8)	17	(5)	23	(7)
Total	184	(100)	180	(100)	135	(100)	152	(100)	314	(100)	332	(100)

appear to be a frequent reason: this is certainly a good sign.

Although these interpretations are bound to be subjective, they seem adequately to express the physicians' self-perception as conscientious but overworked. While, of course, this may be quite true, the patients see the health services in a somewhat different light.

To make a closer assessment of the management of hypertension, 486 patients with previously diagnosed hypertension were selected at random as described in the protocol.

General information on the patients is given in Table 4. Women predominated. Most of the patients had been observed and under care for several years before the survey, with a mean length of observation of 11 years. In most cases, a considerable number of blood pressure measurements were done before treatment began. Patients were seen, on average, at 2.5- to 3-month intervals. At the survey, their average blood pressures were 169/95 mmHg.

A review of the methods used in the diagnostic work-up is one way of assessing patient management. This information is presented in Table 5. Certain features of the outpatient records reviewed are of considerable interest, since they strikingly illustrate some current general medical attitudes, especially in ambulatory medicine. More eye-ground examinations were carried out than family histories taken; more chest X-rays performed than body weights measured. Height was recorded in fewer patients than was post-load blood sugar, and no information was obtained on smoking, alcohol intake and oral contraceptive use. These findings should be interpreted as a reflection of a current general over-reliance on laboratory testing. The spirit

Table 4. Patient survey, Šiška: general information on 486 previously diagnosed hypertensive patients (174 men and 312 women)

Information on patients	Mean	Standard deviation
Total observation period (years)	11	8
Number of blood pressure measurements before treatment began	12	30
Number of readings above 160 mmHg or 95 mmHg	12	28
Number of visits during first year of observation	4	5
Number of visits during last year of observation	5	6
Mean of last three readings of systolic blood pressure (mmHg)	169	21
Mean of last three readings of diastolic blood pressure (mmHg)	95	11

of contemporary medicine should be blamed, rather than the individual physicians.

Treatment methods are summed up in Table 6. Non-drug treatment was prescribed to 80% of all patients with previously diagnosed hypertension. The most common method was sodium restriction, prescribed nevertheless to only 48% of all patients. While 56% (or 273) of all patients were found to be overweight, weight reduction was prescribed to only 39% of all patients, or to 70% of those who were overweight.

At the time of the survey, 80% of the previously diagnosed hypertensives were on drug treatment. Diuretics were prescribed more often than beta-blockers; centrally acting drugs came third. More than one drug was given in 60% of drug therapy.

As stipulated by the protocol, the case histories of the previously diagnosed hypertensives were reviewed, and categorized by the treatment they should have received according to the WHO/ISH guidelines for the management of mild hypertension. According to this standard, 331 patients (68%) were undertreated, as compared with 147 patients (30%) who were treated correctly, while 8 patients (1.6%) were found to be overtreated.

These findings should be considered together with the results of the community survey, presented

Table 5. Patient survey, Šiška: diagnostic work-up given to 486 previously diagnosed hypertensive patients

Procedure	Yes		No		Unknown	
	No.	(%)	No.	(%)	No.	(%)
Was family history taken?	241	(50)	203	(42)	42	(9)
Was body weight measured?	261	(54)	211	(43)	14	(3)
Was height measured?	238	(49)	227	(47)	21	(4)
Was urine analysis done?	395	(81)	87	(18)	4	(1)
Was electrocardiogram taken?	392	(81)	88	(18)	6	(1)
Was serum creatinine done?	232	(48)	127	(26)	127	(26)
Was serum cholesterol done?	303	(62)	103	(21)	80	(16)
Was serum uric acid done?	225	(46)	133	(27)	128	(26)
Was post-load blood sugar done?	340	(70)	96	(20)	50	(10)
Was a chest X-ray taken?	368	(76)	114	(23)	4	(1)
Was eye-ground examination done?	263	(54)	204	(42)	19	(4)

in Table 2. The full extent of undertreatment is shown by the rate of insufficiently treated but diagnosed hypertensives *and* the rate (22%) of unaware hypertensives in the general population. The real picture of overtreatment should be based on the rates of unnecessary treatment given to normotensives (8% with a history of treatment) *and* the seemingly modest 1.6% overtreatment rate in confirmed hypertensives. Although much has been achieved since the rule of halves in the early 1970s, this composite picture shows that much still has to be done at the community level and that action is needed on *both* fronts. Underdiagnosis, unawareness and undertreatment should be corrected, but overdiagnosis and overtreatment may also be a problem.

Consumer Inquiry

Following the protocol, the 486 previously diagnosed hypertensives (174 men and 312 women) were asked to complete anonymously a questionnaire with a few simple questions, placing the patient in the role of the health care consumer. The results are given in Table 7.

Table 6. Patient survey, Šiška: treatment of 486 previously diagnosed hypertensive patients

Treatment	Patients	
	No.	(%)
Non-drug treatment	386	(80)
Weight reduction	191	(39)
Sodium restriction	236	(48)
Physical exercise	184	(38)
Drug treatment	393	(80)
Beta-blockers	127	(26)
Diuretics	146	(30)
Vasodilators	63	(13)
Rauwolfia	39	(8)
Calcium antagonists	36	(7)
Centrally acting antihypertensives	105	(22)
Others	108	(22)

The respondents gave no reply to 6 – 10% of the questions, showing a moderate interest in the inquiry. Nearly 20% of them expressed dissatisfaction with the care they were receiving, and 31% complained about the difficulties of being a patient. About 30% seemed to have difficulties with compliance.

The replies cannot be linked to the respondents, though it might be interesting to see whether negative (or positive) perceptions cluster. A tentative conclusion would be that about a third of the patients have trouble coping with their disease. The questionnaire is too gross to form any firm conclusions. Perhaps the clearest conclusion would be that more attention should be paid to patients' perceptions of their disease and of the care offered them.

Physician Inquiry

An anonymous questionnaire was mailed by the end of 1986 to 950 general practitioners, nearly every one in the Republic of Slovenia. A total of 425 replies were received (a response rate of 45%); of these, 12 replies were invalid. The respondents were 54% male (mean age 43 years) and 46% female (mean age 35 years). The age range was 24 – 75 years. Replies came evenly from all parts of the country.

Table 8 presents the physicians' self-reports on their techniques of blood pressure measurement. Most take blood pressure readings with the patient seated, and select one arm only. They use different cuff sizes in obese people only exceptionally; in

Table 7. Consumer inquiry, Šiška: replies from 486 previously diagnosed hypertensive patients

Question	Answers	Consumers No.	(%)
Is it hard to be a patient with high blood pressure?	No	255	(52)
	Yes	152	(31)
	Hard to say	53	(11)
	No reply	26	(6)
How satisfied are you with the care given for your high blood pressure?	Very satisfied	48	(10)
	Satisfied	279	(57)
	Not satisfied	91	(19)
	Very dissatisfied	2	(–)
	No opinion	23	(5)
	No reply	43	(9)
When was the last time you took drugs for high blood pressure?	Today or yesterday	341	(71)
	2 – 3 days ago	28	(6)
	One week ago	12	(2)
	One week to one month ago	12	(2)
	More than one month ago	43	(9)
	No reply	50	(10)
Do you take your drugs for high blood pressure regularly?	No	128	(26)
	Yes	322	(66)
	No reply	36	(8)
When visiting a clinic, is it important for you to see the same doctor or nurse?	Absolutely	369	(76)
	Rather	58	(12)
	Not especially	25	(5)
	Not at all	1	} (1)
	No opinion	2	
	No reply	31	(6)
Do you usually see the same doctor?	Always	356	(73)
	Often	44	(9)
	Seldom	9	(2)
	Don't know	36	(7)
	No reply	41	(9)

Table 7 (contd)

Question	Answers	Consumers No.	(%)
Occasional deviations in drug taking are quite common. On average, how often during the last month have you missed your tablets (or some of them)?	Never	197	(41)
	Once or twice in the last month	128	(26)
	Once a week	57	(12)
	Several times a week	31	(6)
	Nearly every day	22	(5)
	No reply	51	(10)
Do you think it is easy to remember to take the tablets as prescribed?	No	26	(5)
	Yes	419	(86)
	No reply	41	(9)

fact, only standard cuffs are available on the market. On the other hand, two thirds of the doctors reported using a correction factor in obese patients. A considerable majority use Korotkoff sound phase V, one third measure at a deflation rate of 2 mmHg/second and two thirds take two or more readings at each examination. While 27% of doctors delegate blood pressure measurement to nurses regularly or often, 36% never do so.

As far as instruments are concerned, 87% of doctors use mercury sphygmomanometers; they only exceptionally use automatic devices. Yearly checks of the instrument were reported by 73% and biannual checks by 19% of doctors.

The diagnostic procedures that the general practitioners consider essential for the diagnosis of hypertension are presented in Table 9.

Tables 10 and 11 illustrate the therapeutic attitudes of general practitioners. Practically all of them (95 – 97%) give drug treatment at blood pressure levels above 180/95 mmHg. Most start drug treatment at systolic blood pressure of 160 – 179 mmHg, or diastolic blood pressure of 95 – 114 mmHg. Drug treatment in borderline hypertension (141 – 159/91 – 94 mmHg) is considered necessary by 9 – 11% of physicians (Table 10). The general opinion was that blood pressure can be kept under control with non-drug treatment in about 30% of patients.

The drug preferences of general practitioners are shown in Table 11. A clear difference emerges between the choice of drugs for younger (beta-blockers: 74%) and for elderly patients (diuretics: 48%). Where a long-lasting normalization of blood pressure is achieved, 4% of doctors claimed to discontinue drug treatment often, 28% sometimes and 51% very seldom, and 13% declared they never stop drug therapy.

Doctors considered that their patients' compliance was poor. Most general practitioners claimed that 10 – 50% of patients did not take the prescribed drugs regularly.

About 30% of patients measure their own blood pressure at home. In this group, compliance with drug treatment and blood pressure control seemed to

Table 8. Physician inquiry, Slovenia: reported practices in blood pressure measurement

Question	Answers	Percentage of physicians
Frequency of blood pressure measurement by nurses?	Almost always	6
	Often	21
	Sometimes	37
	Never	36
Arm where the measurement is usually performed?	Left	30
	Right	19
	Either	26
	Both	25
Usual position of the patient at the blood pressure measurement?	Sitting	72
	Supine	16
	Standing	2
	Various	10
Use of different cuff sizes according to the arm circumference?	No	93
	Yes	7
Correction of blood pressure according to the arm circumference?	No	37
	Yes	63
Phase of Korotkoff sound used to measure diastolic blood pressure?	Phase IV	22
	Phase V	78
Deflation rate?	2 mmHg/sec	32
	5 mmHg/sec	48
	10 mmHg/sec	3
	Various	14
	No answer	3
Number of blood pressure readings at each check-up?	One	34
	Two	55
	Three	10
	No answer	1

Table 9. Physician inquiry, Slovenia: diagnostic procedures considered essential for the diagnosis of hypertension

Procedure	Percentage of physicians who use procedure:		
	always	sometimes	never
Urine analysis	87	7	6
Electrocardiogram	83	14	3
Serum potassium	50	34	16
Serum creatinine	77	16	7
Serum cholesterol	76	17	7
Serum uric acid	62	22	16
Blood glucose	79	17	4
Chest X-ray	59	28	13
Eye-ground examination	67	29	4
Intravenous urography	15	69	16
Radionuclide kidney studies	8	65	27
Other	3	29	68

be better. Only 8% of general practitioners kept a register of hypertensive patients. The spread of personal computers may change the present situation.

The general practitioners reported using the following sources of new information in the field of hypertension: medical literature (78%), information from the pharmaceutical industry (74%), professional meetings and special courses (71%), consultation with specialists (47%) and books (23%).

Finally, 25% of physicians declared having checked their own blood pressure in the last month and 49% during the last year, while 18% had had a blood pressure measurement more than a year ago and 8% failed to answer the question; 8% of the respondents were hypertensive themselves.

In conclusion, the inquiry among the general practitioners gave a picture of generally well informed professionals. This seems to be at variance with the pattern of awareness and treatment status shown by the community survey, as shown in Table 2. Further analyses of the various components of health care for hypertension may be useful.

Table 10. Physician inquiry, Slovenia: blood pressure levels at which physicians start drug treatment

Blood pressure level	Physicians who start drug treatment at various blood pressure levels	
	%	Cumulative %
Systolic (mmHg)		
≤ 140	1	1
141 – 159	9	10
160 – 179	71	81
180 – 199	14	95
≥ 200	2	97
No answer	3	100
Diastolic (mmHg)		
≤ 90	1	1
91 – 94	11	12
95 – 114	85	97
115 – 130	1	98
No answer	2	100

Table 11. Physician inquiry, Slovenia: physicians' first choice of drugs

Drug	Percentage of physicians who use various drugs as a first choice in:	
	younger patients	elderly patients
Beta-blockers	74	8
Diuretics	12	48
Vasodilators	4	10
Reserpine	2	4
Calcium antagonists	1	10
Centrally acting antiadrenergic drugs	2	10
ACE inhibitors	0	1
Other	5	9
Total	100	100

7

THE CITY OF VICENZA, ITALY

L. La Vecchia & M. Vincenzi

The project in the city of Vicenza, Italy, included four approaches: a community survey, a patient survey, a consumer inquiry and a physician inquiry. They were carried out in one of the city's districts, though the physician inquiry covered the whole city.

Vicenza has some 112 000 inhabitants and is situated in the north-east of Italy. It is a fairly rich and productive town, with a good number of small and medium-sized industries, commercial activities and well developed agriculture. Social services and health care are provided by the local health unit, which covers the city and the few surrounding settlements and a total of 238 000 people. The city area is administratively divided into seven districts, one of which is the old city centre. As all the others could be considered equivalent one of them, District No. VI, was selected for the study. An additional advantage was that a high degree of cooperation was guaranteed by the local social services. This area includes a highly populated mid-peripheral zone with residential suburbs, business centres, large working-class areas and some rural settlements on the outskirts of the town.

Community Survey

The total population of District No. VI amounts to 27 073 (December 1987). The population aged 35 – 64 years totals 5998 women and 5150 men; of these 2175 women and 1895 men were randomly selected for this study. The 18 general practitioners working in the area were invited to an information meeting, and the local college of physicians endorsed the project as did the health care authorities of the city.

The selected individuals were asked to present themselves at the outpatient clinic of the district for interview and blood pressure checking. Mercury sphygmomanometers, with differential cuff sizes for larger arms, were used.

The composition of the total study population, the random sample drawn, and the sample screened

Collaborators: E. De Dominicis, A. Dell'Anna, R. Fabris, M. Mattiello, L. Novello, M. Sartori & L. Vezu, Division of Clinical Cardiology, Local Health Unit No. 8, University of Verona, Vicenza, Italy. Drs F. Marcolini, F. Carini and L. Florio, clinicians in Vicenza, are acknowledged for their assistance in the investigation.

is given in Table 1. The three age groups were about equally represented. The participation rates were somewhat higher among women than among men, and the rates increased from 65% in the youngest age groups to 75% in the oldest. As seen from the table, a total of 4070 people received a basic questionnaire and invitation letter for a screening examination, and 2854 people attended. Of these, 1010 were re-examined either because of a history of elevated blood pressure, because their blood pressures were elevated at the survey, or because they were currently on hypotensive drug treatment. This rate amounted to 35% of the sample screened – a fairly high figure.

The diagnosis of hypertension should be made only after repeated examinations. The protocol prescribes two re-examinations to exclude transitory blood pressure elevations in those found to be in the hypertensive range at the community survey. Thus, the 1010 people were recalled for a second re-examination. A total of 849 attended the re-examination, a response rate of 84%. This rate may seem satisfactory, but it should be observed that the sample consisted of people who were found to be hypertensive on screening and to whom control measures were offered.

The final results of the community survey (Table 2) refer to those whose blood pressures were measured up to three times, but exclude the 161 suspected hypertensives who dropped out before the last re-examination. Of those ever treated, 14% fell into the normotensive group, 25% into the borderline group and 61% into the hypertensive group. Among those being treated at the time of the examination, 19% were normotensives, 33% were borderline hypertensives and 48% hypertensives. Further, 164 hypertensive and borderline cases (23%) were totally unaware of their condition (51 of these or 31% were borderline hypertensives). As shown in Fig. 1, 215 or 28% of those with confirmed hypertension had a past history of hypertension, with or without previous treatment, but were currently untreated. Of those being treated, blood pressure control was unsatisfactory in 318 and, of these, 41% were borderline. In the other 75 cases who were receiving treatment, blood pressure was normal.

Table 1. Community survey, Vicenza: age and sex composition of study population and samples, and response rate

Age (years)	Study population						Sample drawn					
	Male		Female		Total		Male		Female		Total	
	No.	(%)	No.	(%)	No.	(%)	No.	(%)	No.	(%)	No.	(%)
35 – 44	1 786	(35)	1 924	(32)	3 710	(33)	698	(37)	759	(35)	1 457	(36)
45 – 54	1 733	(34)	2 071	(35)	3 804	(34)	622	(33)	755	(35)	1 377	(34)
55 – 64	1 631	(32)	2 003	(33)	3 634	(33)	575	(30)	661	(30)	1 236	(30)
All ages	5 150	(100)	5 998	(100)	11 148	(100)	1 895	(100)	2 175	(100)	4 070	(100)

Patient Survey

The work-up of the patients with previously diagnosed hypertension was assessed in 656 patients (293 men and 363 women) (Table 3). The medical records were reviewed when they were available, otherwise the patient's statements were used. The following measurements were performed in 47 – 64% of patients: body height and weight, electrocardiogram, urine analysis, blood sugar, serum cholesterol, potassium, creatinine and uric acid; and 43% of patients went through chest X-ray and 29% eye-ground examinations.

Family history and smoking habits were assessed in 61% of patients and alcohol consumption in 58%; 26% of the women were asked about oral contraceptive use. Doctors identified 78% of the overweight patients as overweight.

Individual non-drug measures were recommended to less than half of the patients. Weight reduction was, for example, recommended to only 27% of patients though 78% were regarded as overweight. Low sodium diet and physical exercise were recommended to about 40% of patients, but altogether 74% of the patients received some advice about non-drug treatment.

Table 4 presents the observation period before treatment was started among the 656 previously diagnosed hypertensive patients. In 45% of patients, the observation period was less than 1 week, in 32% it was more than 1 week, while 23% were never treated.

Table 5 presents the number of visits to a physician during the first year after diagnosis, as well as during the last year before the survey. Two thirds of patients had up to six visits during the first year, and the distribution of visits was about the same during the year before the survey.

Drug treatment is shown in Table 6 in the 393 patients already being treated. Diuretics were the most commonly used drugs (65%) followed by ACE inhibitors (29%) and beta-blockers (25%), whereas other drugs were much less commonly used, at least as monotherapy. When two drugs were combined, diuretics and beta-blockers were the most common combination followed by diuretics with

Table 1 (contd)

Age (years)	Sample screened						Response rate		
	Male		Female		Total		Male	Female	Total
	No.	(%)	No.	(%)	No.	(%)	(%)	(%)	(%)
35 – 44	436	(34)	510	(33)	946	(33)	(63)	(67)	(65)
45 – 54	428	(33)	558	(36)	986	(35)	(69)	(74)	(72)
55 – 64	425	(33)	497	(32)	922	(32)	(74)	(75)	(75)
All ages	1 289	(100)	1 565	(100)	2 854	(100)	(68)	(72)	(70)

Table 2. Community survey, Vicenza: awareness and treatment status by blood pressure categories after two re-examinations

Awareness and treatment status	Normotensive			Borderline			Hypertensive			Total	
	No.	% of sample screened	% of normo-tensives	No.	% of sample screened	% of border-lines	No.	% of sample screened	% of hyper-tensives	No.	% of sample screened
Total sample screened[a]	1996	74	100	258	10	100	439	16	100	2693	100
Never told	1873	92	94	51	2	20	113	6	26	2037	100
Told at some time	32	22	2	49	33	19	67	45	15	148	100
Treated at some time	16	14	1	29	25	11	70	61	16	115	100
Treated now	75	19	4	129	33	50	189	48	43	393	100

[a] Minus 161 suspected hypertensives who later dropped out.

ACE inhibitors. Almost all patients (93%) on combination therapy (181 patients or 46% of the total) received diuretics as part of their treatment.

For the group of 164 people in whom hypertension was detected for the first time during the survey, the reasons why the diagnosis was not established earlier were investigated. It was difficult to draw conclusions from these analyses for several reasons. One of the problems was interpreting the frequent discrepancies between blood pressure values perceived by patients as normal and the abnormal values found by the survey. A deeper investigation was carried out in those cases where a satisfactory medical record was available, yet the only solution seemed to be to make a diagnosis of "labile" hypertension in 35 patients (21%). In 29 patients (or 18%) medical control was lacking, and in 43 (or 26%) blood pressure had not been measured during medical visits. A common reason for missing hypertension diagnosis was underestimation, mostly because physicians did not share the same definition of hypertension as the survey team; 36 patients (or 22%) fell into this category.

Consumer Inquiry

A questionnaire was administered to 393 patients under drug treatment at the time of the survey. Table 7 presents the results. Most patients did not experience problems with being a hypertensive patient and most of them were satisfied or very satisfied with the care given. They appeared generally to comply easily with drug therapy; 74% said that they took their drugs regularly and 92% had taken them "today or yesterday". One third of the patients had their blood pressures checked exclusively by their physician.

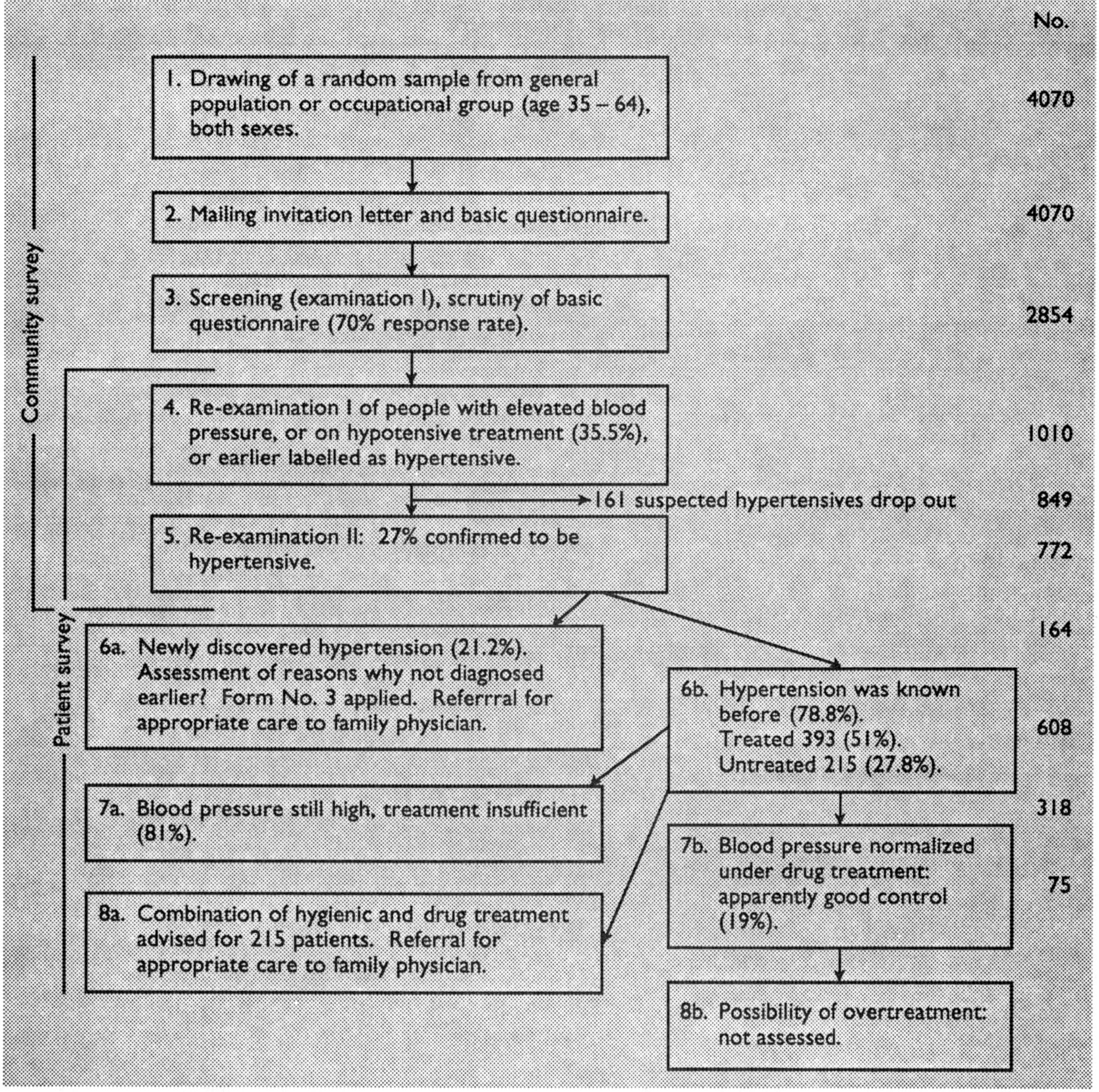

Fig. 1. Community and patient surveys, Vicenza: summary of findings

Table 3. Patient survey, Vicenza: proportion of 656 previously diagnosed hypertensive patients subjected to various procedures

Procedure	Percentage of patients
Clinical work-up	
Body weight	49
Height	47
Urine analysis	63
Electrocardiogram	59
Serum potassium	59
Serum creatinine	60
Serum cholesterol	63
Serum uric acid	59
Blood sugar	64
Oral glucose tolerance test	26
Chest X-ray	43
Eye-ground examination	29
Inquiry about risk factors	
Family history	61
Smoking habits	61
Alcohol consumption	58
Oral contraceptives use	26
Detection of overweight patients	
Patients overweight	47
Overweight patients recognized as such by physician	78
Advice about non-drug measures	
Weight reduction	27
Sodium restriction	39
Physical exercise	43
Non-drug treatment (one or more of the above)	74

Table 4. Patient survey, Vicenza: observation period before drug treatment began in 656 hypertensive patients

Observation period	Percentage of patients
< 1 week	45
1 week – 1 month	22
> 1 month	10
Never treated	23

Table 5. Patient survey, Vicenza: number of visits to a physician during the first year after diagnosis and during the last year before the survey, by 656 hypertensives

Number of visits	Percentage of patients
First year	
None	15
1 – 3	27
4 – 6	17
> 7	35
No information	6
Last year	
None	11
1 – 3	28
4 – 6	21
> 7	35
No information	5

Table 6. Patient survey, Vicenza: drug treatment (as monotherapy or combination therapy) of 393 patients

Drug	Patients No.	(%)
Beta-blockers	100	(25)
Diuretics	255	(65)
Vasodilators	65	(17)
Centrally acting drugs	65	(17)
ACE inhibitors	114	(29)
Other	18	(5)

Of those who had their blood pressure checked by other means, about 60% had it checked at home and 30% at the pharmacy.

Some 78% of the patients considered it absolutely or rather important to see the same doctor at each visit and, in practice, 85% of patients always saw the same doctor for their check-ups.

Physician Inquiry

Questionnaires were sent to every general practitioner in Vicenza, and to the specialists in internal medicine and cardiology working in the area of Vicenza at the time of the community survey (January – June 1988). Of the 248 questionnaires, 135 were sent back (a 54% response rate): of these, 98 were from general practitioners and 37 from hospital specialists. The medical personnel interviewed came from the whole area of Vicenza, not just the District VI used in the community survey. This achieved a sample of sufficient size. Besides, the population of District VI was not necessarily served by the practitioners working in that particular area. The results of the inquiry are presented in Table 8. The vast majority of the physicians personally checked the blood pressure in their patients and without preference for the left or right arm. The patient was generally examined in a sitting position and the blood pressure recorded more than once, with an interval of more than five minutes in 51% of patients. Mercury sphygmomanometers were used most commonly, and the device was standardized once a year by 36%, less often by 57%. Korotkoff V sound was recorded by only 38% of doctors. Only 24% of doctors measured at an accuracy of 2 mmHg.

Over 80% of physicians considered self-measurement valuable and declared they instructed their patients how to do it, while 65% of doctors had had their own blood pressure checked within the last year.

Table 9 shows the handling of patients in the practice. Of the 120 physicians who answered the questions, 58% saw 500 patients or more per year, and 55% saw more than 100 patients with

Table 7. Consumer inquiry, Vicenza: replies from 393 patients under drug treatment

Question	Answers	Percentage of consumers
Is it difficult to be a patient with hypertension?	No	61
	Yes	37
	Hard to say	2
How satisfied are you with the care given?	Very satisfied	12
	Satisfied	69
	Not satisfied	10
	Very dissatisfied	5
	No opinion	4
When did you last take drugs for hypertension?	Today or yesterday	92
	2 – 3 days ago	5
	One week ago	1
	One week to one month ago	2
	More than one month ago	–
	Other, when?	–
Do you take your drugs regularly?	No	26
	Yes	74
Is it important to meet the same doctor?	Absolutely	37
	Rather	41
	Not especially	11
	Not at all	10
	Do not know	1
Do you usually see the same doctor?	Always	85
	Often	12
	Seldom	3
	Never	1
	Do not know	–
Occasional deviations. How often did you miss your drugs last month?	Never	78
	Once or twice in the last month	12
	Once a week	6
	Several times a week	3
	Nearly every day	1
Is it easy to remember your drugs?	No	23
	Yes	77

Table 8. Physician inquiry, Vicenza: reported practices in blood pressure measurement

Reported practices	Percentage of physicians
Measurement taken:	
by physician	88
by nurse	10
by physician or nurse	2
Measurement taken:	
on right arm	17
on left arm	16
on both arms	44
More than one answer	23
Measurement:	
in sitting position	46
in lying position	10
in standing position	9
More than one answer	34
Blood pressure measured:	
only once	14
more than once	86
Interval between readings more than 5 minutes	51
Device used	
mercury	81
aneroid	9
more than one answer	10

Reported practices	Percentage of physicians
Device standardized:	
once a year	36
less often	57
Sounds used	
Korotkoff V	38
Korotkoff IV	47
Values rounded off:	
at 10 mmHg	4
at 5 mmHg	70
at 2 mmHg	24
Self-measurement considered useful	85
Instruction about self-measurement given	81
Physicians' own blood pressure checked:	
less than 6 months ago	48
6 – 12 months ago	17
years ago	29

Table 9. Physician inquiry, Vicenza: information about physicians' practices

Features of the practice	Percentage of physicians
Number of patients seen over past year:[a]	
less than 500	31
500 – 1000	39
over 1000	19
Number of hypertensive patients seen last year:	
less than 100	42
100 or more	55
Practice keeps a register of hypertensive patients	34
Practice has a reminder system	81
Physician thinks personal computer would be useful	61

[a] Each patient counted once only, however many visits.

hypertension per year. Only 34% of the doctors had a special register of hypertensive patients, even though 81% had a reminder system, and 61% thought that a personal computer would be useful for the handling of hypertensive patients.

Table 10 shows the diastolic blood pressure levels that were considered abnormal when the systolic blood pressure was 140 – 159 mmHg. Increasing levels were accepted at increasing ages. In patients under 35 years of age, 90% of physicians thought that diastolic blood pressure of 95 – 99 mmHg was abnormal but, in patients aged 60 or more, only 61% of physicians thought so.

Table 11 shows that somewhat higher blood pressure levels were accepted before treatment is considered necessary. About 90% of physicians would start treatment at diastolic blood pressures of 100 – 104 mmHg in the age groups below 35 and 35 – 59, while in patients aged 60 or more 90% of physicians would start at levels of 105 – 109 mmHg.

Table 12 shows that 80% of physicians take three or more blood pressure measurements before making a diagnosis of hypertension, and the interval between subsequent controls is usually one week.

Table 13 shows that non-drug treatment was widely recommended to patients, and assessment of risk factors was also extensive. According to the

Table 10. Physician inquiry, Vicenza: diastolic blood pressure levels physicians consider abnormal (when systolic blood pressure is 140 – 159 mmHg)

Diastolic blood pressure (mmHg)	Cumulative percentage of physicians who consider various blood pressure levels as abnormal in patients aged:		
	< 35 years	35 – 59 years	60 + years
< 90	9	2	1
90 – 94	66	34	18
95 – 99	90	81	61
100 – 104	98	99	96
105 – 109	98	99	97
> 110	98	99	99
No answer (%)	2	1	1

Table 11. Physician inquiry, Vicenza: diastolic blood pressure levels at which physicians consider treatment necessary (when systolic blood pressure is 140 – 159 mmHg)

Diastolic blood pressure (mmHg)	Cumulative percentage of physicians who consider treatment necessary at various blood pressure levels in patients aged:		
	< 35 years	35 – 59 years	60 + years
< 90	1	1	1
90 – 94	21	14	7
95 – 99	60	50	32
100 – 104	91	90	79
105 – 109	92	94	89
> 110	93	95	96
No answer (%)	7	5	4

Table 12. Physician inquiry, Vicenza: method of diagnosis

Method	Percentage of physicians
Number of blood pressure measurements taken before diagnosis	
one	0
two	15
three or more	81
Time interval between subsequent measurements	
one day	7
one week	63
one month	21

Table 13. Physician inquiry, Vicenza: attitudes towards non-drug therapy as reflected by actions reported by physicians

Reported action	Percentage of physicians
Advise non-drug treatment	97
weight reduction	99
sodium restriction	95
physical exercise	90
behavioural therapy	56
stopping oral contraception	58
Assess cardiovascular disease risk factors	
smoking	99
hyperlipidaemia	94
alcohol consumption	93

Table 14. Physician inquiry, Vicenza: procedures performed in the clinical work-up of hypertensive patients

Procedure	Percentage of physicians
Body weight	93
Height	51
Urine analysis	95
Electrocardiogram	94
Serum potassium	96
Serum creatinine	96
Serum cholesterol	96
Serum uric acid	90
Post-load blood sugar	33
Blood urea nitrogen	93
Chest X-ray	79
Eye-ground examination	86

Table 15. Physician inquiry, Vicenza: physicians' preferences for first choice drugs

Drug	Percentage of physicians who use various drugs as a first choice in patients aged:					
	< 35 years		35 – 59 years		60 + years	
	Male	Female	Male	Female	Male	Female
Beta-blockers	42	41	16	16	1	0
Diuretics	8	14	17	18	25	24
Vasodilators	0	0	3	1	1	1
Calcium antagonists	1	1	26	24	20	21
ACE inhibitors	6	15	26	24	20	21
Combinations	7	20	29	28	28	27
Other	0	0	1	1	1	1
No answer	2	10	4	7	6	8

patients' survey, however, there were considerably lower figures for these interventions.

Most of the diagnostic procedures indicated in the questionnaire were said to be performed by 90% or more of physicians (Table 14). Measurement of height and oral glucose tolerance tests were less commonly performed (51% and 33%, respectively). Table 15 shows physicians' preferences for first choice drugs. Beta-blockers were commonly used among younger patients but rarely in those aged over 60. The use of diuretics increased somewhat with age. In the age range 35 – 59, ACE inhibitors, calcium antagonists and a combination of drugs were commonly used as a first line, and physicians used similar prescriptions in the older age group. Just over 50% of physicians reduce the drug after normalization, but only 2% discontinue drug treatment altogether.

The physicians' general attitudes towards hypertension control are shown in Table 16. Most physicians felt that the media can play a potentially supportive role in the management of hypertensive patients. Many physicians considered the side effects of antihypertensive drugs as the price that patients must pay for the normalization of their blood pressure.

Information on hypertension and cardiovascular risk factors was generally obtained through medical journals, continuing education programmes, textbooks and the pharmaceutical industry, whereas leagues against hypertension and national hypertension education programmes were of very little importance.

Table 16. Physician inquiry, Vicenza: physicians' general attitudes towards hypertension control

Question	Answers	Percentage of physicians
Is there sufficient coverage from the news media regarding hypertension:		
on television?	Yes	45
	No	48
on radio?	Yes	36
	No	47
in newspapers?	Yes	47
	No	44
Is there support from the media for the treatment of hypertension?	Yes	73
	No	24
Are patients negatively affected psychologically by continued treatment?	Yes	34
	No	63
Should side effects be accepted or tolerated by the patients?	Yes	59
	No	38
How do you usually obtain information on hypertension and other cardiovascular risk factors?	Medical journals	84
	Continuing education programmes	64
	Textbooks	60
	Pharmaceutical industry information	58
	Television/radio/newspapers	3
	Leagues against hypertension	1
	WHO	13
	National hypertension education programmes	4
	Other	8

8

TWO INDUSTRIAL POPULATIONS IN ROMANIA

C. Carp, I. David, G. Nandris, G. Calangiu, D. Enachescu, I. Coman, E. Apetrei, I. Stoian & C. Ginghina

Two industrial populations were selected in Romania for a community survey, a patient survey, a consumer inquiry and a physician inquiry: workers in the aluminium factory in Slatina and in the machine factory in Sibiu.

These industrial populations may not be representative of the general population of Romania, which has been shown to have an 8 – 15% prevalence of arterial hypertension in various areas.[a] Nevertheless, these industrial plants are typical of the country's heavy industry with regard to the organization of the health services, the health problems and the quality of health care.

Community and Patient Surveys

Slatina is a medium-size town some 200 km west of Bucharest, the country's capital. The aluminium factory has nearly 23 000 workers. Aluminium is produced by electrolysis and heavy parts for machines are manufactured in the foundry. The workers are mostly men; they are of mixed, urban and rural origin, and some 10% still commute between village and factory.

Sibiu is one of the bigger provincial cities of Romania, in the region of Transylvania, with about 180 000 inhabitants, some 300 km north-west of Bucharest. Unlike in Slatina, the working population is composed of traditional workers, almost exclusively of urban origin. There are slightly more men than women. The factory manufactures parts for cars, textile machines and various instruments, and is midway between heavy and light industry. It has about 15 000 workers.

The population of both factories has been roughly divided into two age groups: 16 – 34 years and 35 – 64 years. The retirement age is 65 years, and thus the upper age limit of the individuals studied. The lower age limit of employment is 16 years and

[a] Steinbach, M. et al. The Bucharest multifactorial prevention trial of coronary heart disease – ten year follow up: 1971 – 1982. *Revue roumaine de médecine interne*, **22**(2): 99 – 106 (1984).

a considerable proportion of the workers belonged to the younger age group. Figures for the total population are presented in Table 1.

The findings for the age group 35 – 64 in both Slatina and Sibiu are summarized in Fig. 1. From the total of 17 334 people, a sample of 9774 men and women was drawn. As the workers were examined in the dispensary of the factory itself, there were no non-responders. Although at initial screening the proportion of possible hypertensives was rather high (27.6%), the percentage of individuals with hypertension confirmed at the second re-examination fell to 6.2% of the sample. This is rather low compared to the prevalence rates in the general population, because many unhealthy people are excluded from industrial populations owing to initial selection procedures or early retirement (the so-called "healthy worker" effect).

Despite the systematic health examinations carried out each year in the factories, however, 112 new cases of hypertension were found, i.e. 1.2% of the total sample or 18% of the individuals with confirmed hypertension. Conversely, 82% of the hypertensive subjects had been aware of their condition before the screening. Such a rate of awareness would be satisfactory if found in a general population, but should be considered insufficient for an industrial population under stricter health control.

The treatment status of the previously diagnosed 494 hypertensive patients was analysed, as described in the protocol. Insufficient treatment was found in 53% of the known hypertensives, against apparently good control in 47% of the cases – a finding similar to the old rule of the halves. Furthermore, in 5% of the cases, the patient was probably overtreated or treated unnecessarily.

In conclusion, the existence of factory health services and of systematic health examinations is not in itself a guarantee of optimal control of hypertension in a particular population.

One way of assessing the level of medical care is to review the methods used in the clinical work-up. Table 2 presents such a review in 341 patients (202 men and 139 women). Although the mere fact that a test has been performed does not tell whether and how its results were used in the diagnostic process, underrepresented items are less likely and missing items obviously unlikely to have been used. On the other hand, procedures performed very often are also unlikely to have been fully used. Smoking habits or alcohol consumption were recorded in 33 – 35% of patients, while an electrocardiogram

Table 1. Community survey, Romania: age and sex composition of two factory populations

Age (years)	Population								
	Slatina			Sibiu			Slatina + Sibiu		
	Male	Female	Total	Male	Female	Total	Male	Female	Total
16 – 34	8 105	4 149	12 254	4 716	3 399	8 115	12 821	7 548	20 369
35 – 64	7 851	2 734	10 585	4 007	2 742	6 749	11 858	5 476	17 334
All ages (16 – 64)	15 956	6 883	22 839	8 731	6 141	14 864	24 679	13 024	37 703

Fig. 1. Community and patient surveys, Romania: summary of findings

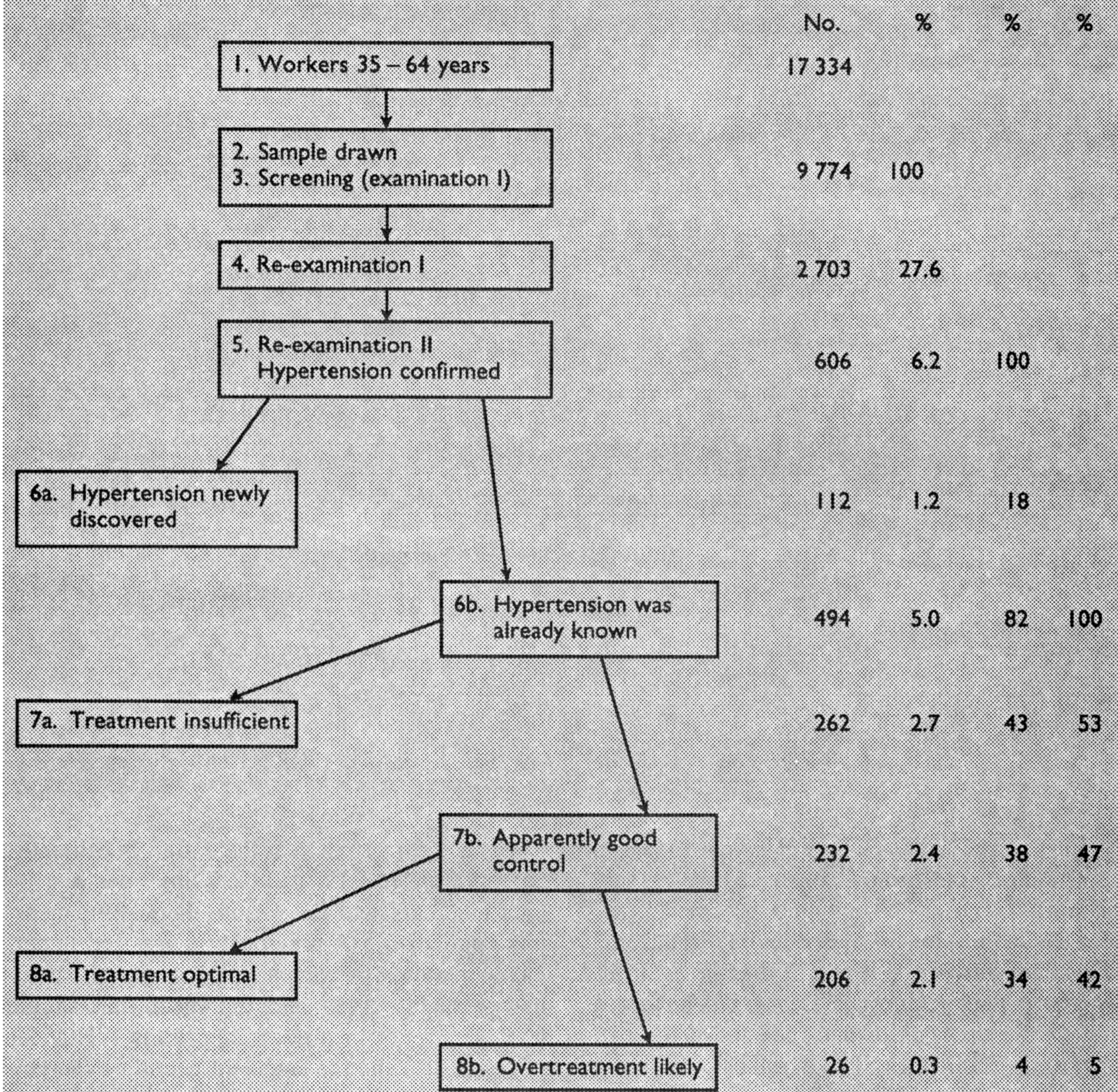

Table 2. Patient survey, Romania: clinical work-up given to 341 previously diagnosed hypertensive patients

Procedure	Yes No.	(%)
Was family history taken?	321	(94)
Was body weight measured?	328	(96)
Was height measured?	326	(96)
Was urine analysis done?	334	(98)
Was electrocardiogram taken?	335	(98)
Was serum creatinine analysed?	256	(75)
Was serum cholesterol analysed?	314	(92)
Was serum uric acid analysed?	103	(30)
Was post-load blood sugar test performed?	19	(6)
Was chest X-ray taken?	313	(92)
Was eye-ground examination made?	241	(70)
Is smoking habit of patient recorded?	114	(33)
Is alcohol intake recorded?	121	(35)

was performed in 98%, chest X-ray in 92% and eye-ground examination in 70% of all cases. A safe assumption seems to be that these proportions are more an expression of the doctors' traditional values than of the real needs of disease management. Considerable differences emerged, however, between the methods of management of the two populations studied. In Slatina, the patients saw a doctor or nurse on average 24 times in the first year and 12 times per year thereafter. In Sibiu, the patients were seen on average 7 times per year.

Table 3 presents the various therapeutic measures applied to 511 previously diagnosed hypertensive patients. A comparison between the treatment actually given and treatment that should have been prescribed according to the WHO/ISH guidelines for the management of mild hypertension helped to categorize patients into the well

Table 3. Patient survey, Romania: treatment of 511 hypertensive patients

Treatment	Patients No.	(%)
Non-drug treatment	289	(57)
weight reduction	84	(16)
sodium restriction	289	(57)
physical exercise	92	(18)
Drug treatment instituted immediately	236	(46)
beta-blockers	146	(29)
diuretics	165	(32)
vasodilators	50	(10)
rauwolfia	34	(7)
calcium antagonists	39	(8)
centrally acting drugs	20	(4)
others (mainly ACE inhibitors)	54	(11)

treated, overtreated and undertreated groups in Fig. 1.

Non-drug treatment was instituted in 57% of the patients. This consisted in most cases of advice to moderate salt intake. A low proportion of patients was considered overweight (93 or 18%). This may be explained by the very often heavy physical work of the subjects. Weight reduction, therefore, played only a secondary role in this particular population. Obviously, the same applies to physical exercise as a therapeutic measure.

Drug treatment was instituted immediately, without first trying out non-drug therapy, in 46% of the cases. The most commonly used drugs were diuretics, followed by beta-blockers. Vasodilators, rauwolfia and calcium antagonists were given less often.

Consumer Inquiry

How the patients themselves perceived the treatment they were receiving is presented in Table 4. The simple questionnaire described in the protocol was given to 341 patients under treatment (202 men and 139 women). The results of such an inquiry, even if anonymous, should be taken with caution, when coming from a highly dependent population such as factory workers examined in the health care facilities of the factory where they are employed. Only 13% said that they were not satisfied with the

Table 4. Consumer inquiry, Romania: replies from 341 previously diagnosed hypertensive patients

Question	Answers	Consumers No.	(%)
Is it hard to be a patient with high blood pressure?	No	42	(12)
	Yes	231	(68)
	Hard to say	68	(20)
How satisfied are you with the care given for your high blood pressure?	Very satisfied	119	(35)
	Satisfied	177	(52)
	Not satisfied	27	(8)
	Very dissatisfied	0	
	No opinion	18	(5)
When was the last time you took drugs for high blood pressure?	Today or yesterday	129	(38)
	2 – 3 days ago	44	(13)
	One week ago	51	(15)
	One week to one month ago	39	(11)
	More than one month ago	78	(23)
Do you take your drugs for high blood pressure regularly?	No	140	(41)
	Yes	201	(59)
When visiting a clinic, is it important for you to see the same doctor or nurse?	Absolutely	104	(30)
	Rather	111	(33)
	Not especially	69	(20)
	Not at all	45	(13)
	No opinion	12	(4)
Do you usually see the same doctor?	Always	119	(35)
	Often	138	(40)
	Seldom	75	(22)
	Never	9	(3)
Occasional deviations in drug taking are quite common. On average, how often during the last month have you missed your tablets (or some of them)?	Never	126	(37)
	Once or twice in the last month	86	(25)
	Once a week	39	(11)
	Several times a week	48	(14)
	Nearly every day	42	(12)
Do you think it is easy to remember to take the tablets as prescribed?	No	120	(35)
	Yes	221	(65)

care given or had no opinion on it, although 68% complained that "it is hard to be a patient with high blood pressure".

Drug taking did not seem to be regular. Only 38% of the patients said they had taken their medication the same day or the day before answering the questionnaire, but 59% thought they were taking their drugs regularly. This fact is most probably due to a lack of communication between doctors and patients. It is also in keeping with the rather mitigated need the patients felt to be seen regularly by the same doctor (30%).

In conclusion, despite the weaknesses of the questionnaire, certain lessons for future improvement of medical care can be derived from this consumer inquiry.

Physician Inquiry

A questionnaire was sent to 115 physicians in Sibiu and Slatina, mostly general practitioners but also some internists and cardiologists. Within a week, 98 physicians (85%) had returned the questionnaire. The results are given in the summary Tables 8 – 13 in Chapter 3 and present a positive self-image of the responders. Thus, for example, 83% declared measuring blood pressure on both arms; 93% asserted having a register and 92% a reminder system for their hypertensive patients; 99% recommended weight reduction to their patients; and 98% said they did eyeground examinations. These figures confirm that the surveyed physicians were aware of the standards of good medical practice and should be seen as an expression of their wish to comply with these standards.

9

THE TOWN OF SIANO, NEAR NAPLES, ITALY

V. Canonico, L. Forgione & F. Rengo

The project in the town of Siano, Italy, consisted of a community survey, a patient survey, a consumer inquiry and a physician inquiry.

Siano is a little town 32 km from Naples. Most of the inhabitants are farmers, with arable farming the main activity. Siano has few public and private clinics, and no hospitals. The closest is 16 km away and has four departments: cardiology, general medicine, surgery and obstetrics.

Community Survey

The total population of Siano comprises 2840 men and 3505 women. The age group 35 – 64 included 3842 individuals. Of these, 1462 men and 1727 women were screened, giving a response rate of 83%.

The results are given in Table 1. Of the total sample of 3189 people screened, 765 (or 24%) were confirmed to be in the hypertensive range after two re-examinations. Of these hypertensives, 410 (or 61%) were under treatment, 168 (or 22%) had a history of hypertension but were not treated, and 260 (or 34%) were newly discovered. Of those on treatment, 53% had borderline or normal blood pressure levels, whereas 47% still had blood pressure levels above 140/90 mmHg.

A summary of these findings indicates the high prevalence of hypertension in the area, with a relatively low awareness of the condition and a rather high blood pressure level in spite of treatment. Overtreatment did not appear to be a problem.

Patient Survey

The methods used in the clinical work-up of 410 previously diagnosed patients is given in Table 2. Body weight was measured in only 35% of patients and height in 18%, and eye-ground examinations were performed in 11%. On the other hand, urine analyses and blood sugar measurements were performed in just over 60% of patients, and electrocardiograms and chest X-rays in just over 50%, whereas serum cholesterol was measured in less than a third as were serum potassium, serum creatinine and serum uric acid. Family history and smoking habits were assessed in about two thirds of patients but alcohol intake in only

Table 1. Community survey, Siano: awareness and treatment status after two re-examinations

Awareness and treatment status	Male			Female			Total		
	No.	% of sample screened	% of hyper-tensives	No.	% of sample screened	% of hyper-tensives	No.	% of sample screened	% of hyper-tensives
Total sample screened	1462	100	–	1727	100	–	3189	100	–
Total found hypertensive	344	24	100	421	24	100	765	24	100
Never told	114	8	33	146	9	35	260	8	34
Told at some time	230	16	67	275	16	65	505	16	66
Treated at some time	148	10	43	189	11	45	337	11	44
Treated now	180	12	52	230	13	55	410	13	61

about a third. Overweight was detected in about two thirds of hypertensives.

Weight reduction, low sodium diet and physical exercise were recommended to a relatively low percentage of patients, but altogether about half of the patients were regarded as getting some type of non-drug treatment.

The drugs used are listed in Table 3, showing that 45% of patients received diuretics, 15% beta-blockers and 15% calcium antagonists.

Consumer Inquiry

The 410 previously diagnosed and treated hypertensive patients were asked to complete anonymously a questionnaire with a few simple questions, in which they were considered as consumers of health care (Table 4). Nearly 60% of the patients were not satisfied or very dissatisfied with the care given, and 15% had no opinion; 40% considered it difficult to be a patient with hypertension; 70% took their drugs regularly, and 32% said that they had missed taking their drugs once or twice in the last months. About two thirds considered it easy to remember to take their drugs; 88% always saw the same doctor and 82% considered it very important to meet the same doctor regularly.

Physician Inquiry

A questionnaire was sent to every general practitioner in Siano. Replies were received from 126 (a 72% response rate). They saw an average of 560 patients each year of whom nearly 16% were hypertensive. The responses to the questionnaires are seen in Tables 5 – 8. Nurses measure the blood pressure in only 10% of cases. It is measured on both arms by only 5% of physicians or nurses and by nearly half of the respondents on patients in the lying position. Mercury devices were used by 75% of respondents

Table 2. Patient survey, Siano: proportion of 410 previously diagnosed hypertensive patients subjected to various procedures

Procedure	Percentage of patients
Clinical work-up	
Body weight	35
Height	18
Urine analysis	62
Electrocardiogram	54
Serum potassium	32
Serum creatinine	30
Serum cholesterol	27
Serum uric acid	32
Blood sugar	65
Oral glucose tolerance test	37
Chest X-ray	55
Eye-ground examination	11
Inquiry about risk factors	
Family history	61
Smoking habits	75
Alcohol consumption	38
Oral contraceptives use	14
Detection of overweight patients	
Patients overweight	62
Overweight patients recognized as such by physician	70
Advice about non-pharmacological measures	
Weight reduction	20
Sodium restriction	30
Physical exercise	10
Non-drug treatment (one or more of the above)	52

Table 3. Patient survey, Siano: drug treatment (as monotherapy or combination therapy) of 410 previously diagnosed hypertensive patients

Drug	Percentage of patients
Beta-blockers	15
Diuretics	45
Rauwolfia	5
Calcium antagonists	15
Centrally acting sympathicolytics	5
ACE inhibitors	15

and very few used automatic devices. Over 70% of physicians standardized the devices once every second year and 80% read blood pressures to the nearest 5 mmHg; 60% of physicians thought that self-measurement was useful and 40% declared that they were teaching self-measurement to their patients.

Drug treatment was considered necessary at systolic blood pressures above 150, 160 and 180 mmHg respectively in the age groups below 35, 35 – 59 and 60 years and above (Table 6).

Non-drug treatment is advised by 88% of physicians and cardiovascular disease risk factors are assessed by up to 99% (Table 7).

Table 8 displays the clinical work-up considered important by the physicians. Measurement of body weight, urine analysis, electrocardiogram, serum cholesterol and blood glucose were performed by 80% or more of physicians. Serum creatinine and serum uric acid were measured by only about 50% and eye-ground examination by 32% of physicians. Nearly 70% performed an X-ray.

The preferences of physicians for the various drug families were as follows: beta-blockers for patients under 35 years of age, diuretics for those aged 35 – 59 years, and ACE inhibitors or calcium antagonists for those over 60 years. Just over 80% of physicians tried reducing the dosage when pressure was normalized.

Table 9 shows that the usual sources of information about the work-up and treatment of hypertensive patients were medical journals and information from the pharmaceutical industry, whereas as few as 21% got their information through national programmes.

Table 4. Consumer inquiry, Siano: replies from 410 previously diagnosed hypertensive patients

Question	Answers	Percentage of consumers
Is it difficult to be a patient with hypertension?	No	50
	Yes	40
	Hard to say	10
How satisfied are you with the care given?	Very satisfied	8
	Satisfied	18
	Not satisfied	38
	Very dissatisfied	21
	No opinion	15
When did you last take drugs for hypertension?	Today or yesterday	89
	2 – 3 days ago	7
	One week ago	3
	One week to one month ago	1
	More than one month ago	0
	Other	0
Do you take your drugs regularly?	No	30
	Yes	70
Is it important to meet the same doctor?	Absolutely	82
	Rather	15
	Not especially	3
	Not at all	0
	Do not know	0
Do you usually see the same doctor?	Always	88
	Often	10
	Seldom	2
	Never	0
	Do not know	0
Occasional deviations. How often did you miss your drugs last month?	Never	53
	Once or twice in the last month	32
	Once a week	8
	Several times a week	5
	Nearly every day	2
Is it easy to remember your drugs?	No	34
	Yes	66

Table 5. Physician inquiry, Siano: reported practices in blood pressure measurement

Reported practices	Percentage of physicians
Blood pressure measured by nurses	10
Blood pressure measured:	
in right arm	38
in left arm	22
in both arms	5
in sitting position	27
in lying position	45
in standing position	4
Interval between blood pressure measurements at least 5 minutes	31
Blood pressure measuring device	
mercury	75
automatic	2
aneroid	23
Instrument standardized:	
once a year	22
once in two years	72
Diastolic reading based on:	
Korotkoff IV	18
Korotkoff V	82
Values recorded to the next:	
10 mmHg	14
5 mmHg	80
2 mmHg	6
Physician thinks self-measurement is useful	60
Physician teaches self-measurement to patients	40
Physician checked own blood pressure during past year	68

Table 6. Physician inquiry, Siano: blood pressure most physicians define as hypertension and at which most start drug treatment

Age of patient	Blood pressure (mmHg): that most physicians define as hypertension		Blood pressure (mmHg): at which most physicians start drug treatment	
	systolic	diastolic	systolic	diastolic
Under 35 years	140	90	150	95
35 – 59 years	150	90	160	95
60 years and over	160	90	180	100

Table 7. Physician inquiry, Siano: attitudes towards non-drug therapy as reflected by actions reported by physicians

Reported action	Percentage of physicians
Advise non-drug treatment	88
weight reduction	80
sodium restriction	82
physical exercise	61
stopping oral contraception	78
Assess cardiovascular disease risk factors	
smoking	97
hyperlipidaemia	99
alcohol consumption	93
diabetes	90
hyperuricaemia	37

Table 8. Physician inquiry, Siano: procedures performed in the clinical work-up of hypertensive patients

Procedure	Percentage of physicians
Body weight	80
Height	40
Urine analysis	83
Electrocardiogram	92
Serum potassium	43
Serum creatinine	51
Serum cholesterol	90
Serum uric acid	51
Blood glucose	80
Post-load blood sugar	32
Chest X-ray	68
Eye-ground examination	32

Table 9. Physician inquiry, Siano: usual sources of information on hypertension

Information source	Percentage of physicians
Medical journals	90
Continuing education programmes	20
Textbooks	18
Pharmaceutical industry	92
Television/radio/newspapers	32
Antihypertensive leagues	–
WHO	–
ISH	–
National programmes	–
Congresses	21

10

HYPERTENSION DETECTION AND FOLLOW-UP PROGRAMME IN ASHKELON, ISRAEL

R.J. Viskoper, L. Bregman, J. Mishal, S. Oren, M. Klier, A. Laszt, D. Pinkesfeld & E. Klier

In the town of Ashkelon, Israel, a community survey, a patient survey, a consumer inquiry and a physician inquiry were carried out.

A community-wide hypertension detection and follow-up programme was started in Ashkelon, Israel, in 1980 by the Barzilai Medical Centre, in cooperation with the Community Centre for the Prevention of Cardiovascular Diseases. Under the programme, a health examination takes place, by invitation, at the worksite or at a community health centre. Blood pressure, height, weight, smoking habits and family history of cardiovascular diseases, diabetes and hypertension are recorded; the information is scored; and those considered at high risk are referred to a clinic for the prevention of cardiovascular diseases. This part of the Hypertension Management Audit Project took place in the context of this programme.

Ashkelon is a town of 52 000 inhabitants, situated 56 km south of Tel Aviv on the eastern shore of the Mediterranean Sea. The settlement is of ancient origin, built on the remains of an old biblical Philistine town, but is at present a modern industrial city with several factories and a port. The population is predominantly of North African origin, with a smaller segment of European and South African Jews. Virtually the total population is under health insurance by the Kupat Holim, the General Federation of Labour's General Sick Fund; Barzilai Medical Centre, too, belongs to the Sick Fund.

Community and Patient Survey

Up to the time of writing this report, 11 000 people aged 35 to 64 were screened, amounting to about one third of the town's population of that age. Some 90% were blue collar employees of factories; about 70% were of Sephardic origin. From these surveyed people, 3500 aged 35 to 64 years were selected at random by the Medical Centre's statistical service for inclusion in the Hypertension Management Audit Project. Thus, unlike in other populations participating in the Project, the Ashkelon Audit took place in an environment with an organized hypertension community control programme that had been under way for several years.

Out of the sample, 3012 people were examined (an 86% response rate). Among these, 307 (10%) had elevated blood pressure (about 160 or 90 mmHg) at the initial examination done in the context of the original community programme (Fig. 1). These people were re-examined on two further occasions, and 162 individuals were eventually retained as having persistent high blood pressure. Together with those who had earlier been found to be in the hypertensive range and actually had normal blood pressure owing to treatment, definite hypertension was found to have an overall prevalence of 7% in the age group 35 to 64 years. Of these, only 6% were unaware of their condition, and a total of 18% were untreated – a favourable health care situation explained by the fact that the hypertension control programme in this community had been operating five years before the present survey began.

Although hypertension increases considerably with age, this sample showed no great difference

Fig. 1. Community survey, Ashkelon: summary of findings

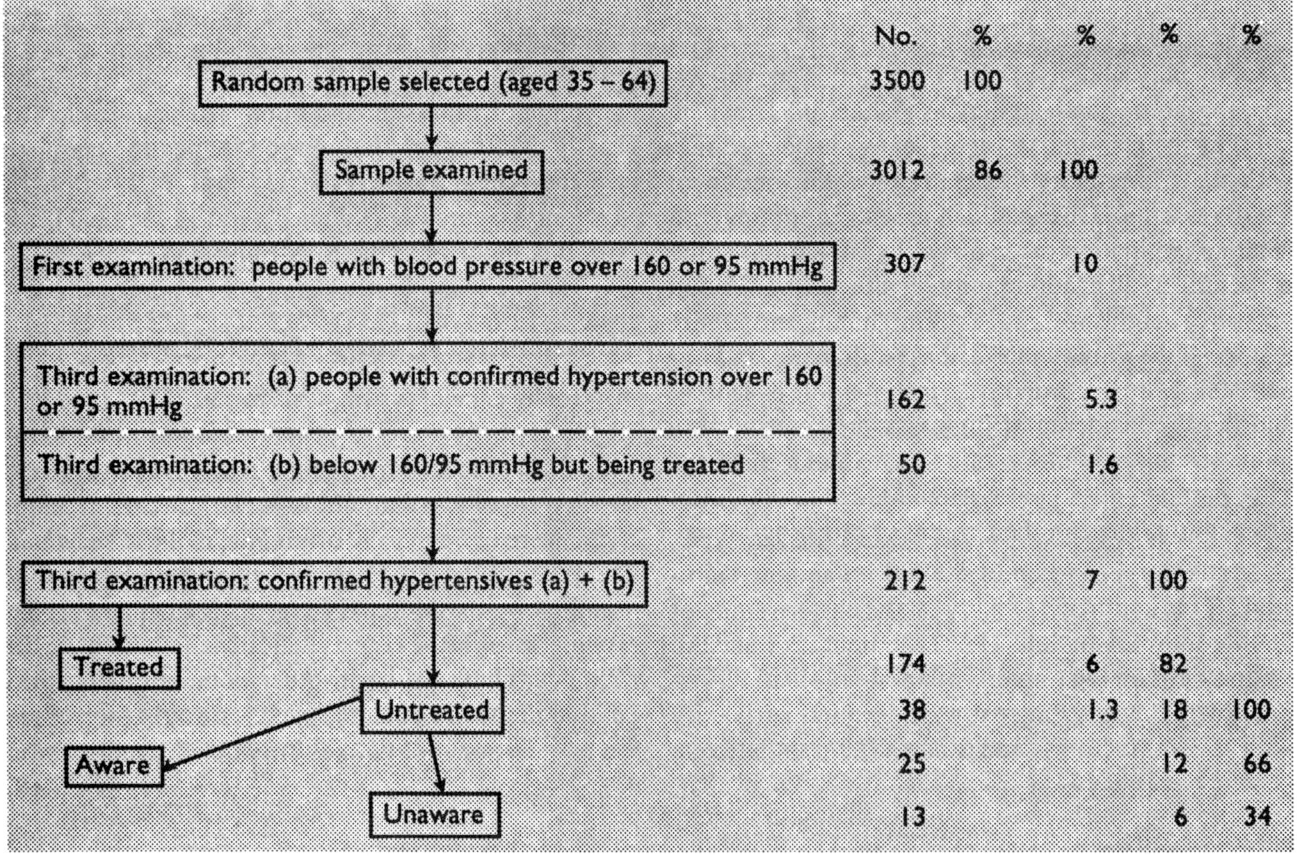

between the younger and older age groups: 45% were between 35 and 49 years old, while 55% were aged 50 to 64 years. Women (55%) predominated slightly over men (45%).

As may have been expected in such a population, serum lipid values were high, with a serum cholesterol concentration of 227 (± 43) mg/dl in men and 235 (± 48) mg/dl in women; mean serum triglycerides were 175 (± 105) mg/dl in men and 153 (± 77) mg/dl in women. Some 5% of the hypertensives had serum cholesterol values above 300 mg/dl. The proportion of heavy smokers was surprisingly low: only 5% smoked more than 20 cigarettes per day. On the other hand, overweight was very common. More than half the hypertensives were more than 20% over the ideal body weight, and almost one third (29%) were more than 30% over the ideal weight. This is in striking contrast with the favourable picture as regards awareness and treatment status.

By the same token, the practice of health care showed surprising insufficiencies. Out of a sample of 147 previously diagnosed hypertensives (Table 1), 28% were not examined in the three months preceding the survey, and 84% were not examined in the preceding month. These figures show that follow-up of hypertensive patients usually occurs at rather long intervals. In addition, blood pressure had not been measured in 20% of those who had been examined. Only 52% of the subjects had received any information about their blood pressure.

Consumer Inquiry

According to the consumer inquiry (Table 2), the doctor – patient relationship does not seem to be very close. Some 19% of patients declared that it is not especially (or not at all) important for them to see the same doctor or nurse on each visit; only slightly more than half the patients (55%) felt that it

Table 1. Patient survey, Ashkelon: quality and timing of last examination of 147 previously diagnosed hypertensive patients

Question	Answers	Patients No.	(%)
When was the last examination performed?	Less than a month ago	23	(16)
	1 – 3 months ago	96	(65)
	More than 3 months ago	28	(19)
Was blood pressure measured?	No	29	(20)
	Yes	112	(76)
	Don't remember	6	(4)
Were blood pressure values told to patient?	No	54	(37)
	Yes	77	(52)
	Don't remember	16	(11)

Table 2. Consumer inquiry, Ashkelon: replies from 147 previously diagnosed hypertensive patients

Question	Answers	Consumers No.	Consumers (%)
When visiting a clinic, is it important for you to meet the same doctor or nurse?	Absolutely	81	(55)
	Rather	36	(24)
	Not especially	28	(19)
	Not at all	1	(1)
	No opinion	1	(1)
Do you always see the same doctor?	Always	95	(64)
	Often	52	(36)
How often have you missed your tablets during the last month?	Never	70	(48)
	Once or twice	61	(41)
	Once a week	6	(4)
	Several times per week	3	(2)
	Don't know	7	(5)
Is it easy to remember to take the tablets as prescribed?	No	53	(36)
	Yes	94	(64)
Is it difficult to be a patient with high blood pressure?	No	54	(37)
	Yes	84	(57)
	Hard to say	9	(6)
How satisfied are you with the care given for your high blood pressure?	Very satisfied	46	(31)
	Satisfied	60	(41)
	Not satisfied	28	(19)
	Very dissatisfied	3	(2)
	No opinion	10	(7)
When was the last time you took drugs for high blood pressure?	Today or yesterday	134	(90)
	2 – 3 days ago	11	(8)
	One week ago	1	(1)
	One week to one month ago	1	(1)
Do you take your drugs regularly?	No	17	(12)
	Yes	130	(88)

was very important for them to see the same doctor all the time. Actually, 64% did see the same doctor on each occasion.

On the other hand, almost half of the patients (48%) declared not having missed a single tablet during the past month, while 41% admitted only having missed one or two tablets during this period. Barely 2% admitted missing medication several times a week.

Few patients expressed strong dissatisfaction with the health care they received but, on the other hand, only 72% seemed to be really satisfied with the health services. The overall picture is thus a complex one, as may have been expected. On the other hand, in view of the crudeness of the instrument used, only a sketchy impression of the situation could be obtained. A further, more elaborate analysis of the care provider/consumer relationships would nevertheless be justified.

Physician Inquiry

The physician inquiry questionnaire was addressed to 30 general practitioners in the Ashkelon area. All of them had been involved in the community programme. The results are presented in Tables 3 – 9.

The self-portrait of the physicians is favourable, as expected, indicating that they are well aware of what *should* be done (Table 3). All physicians use mercury sphygmomanometers, and are well aware of the need to check them periodically. The majority surprisingly declare using Korotkoff IV phase sounds. The average 10.7-minute pause between the two blood pressure readings seems to be a curious overstatement.

The physicians seem to be very busy, but only 6% of their patients are hypertensive (Table 4). Nevertheless, they keep a register of hypertensive patients, and most of them use a reminder system. The physicians' prevailing concepts of the definition of hypertension are given in Table 5. They are clearly age-related, more so than the WHO recommendations.

Non-drug treatment is being advised at least in theory. Weight reduction, for example, may be advised but a high proportion of patients is still overweight.

Physicians assert using a broad spectrum of diagnostic tests on their hypertensive patients, including a chest X-ray and post-load blood sugar test (Table 7). Beta-blockers and diuretics are the first choice single drugs, but various combinations are mentioned in a greater proportion than monotherapy as first choice treatment (Table 8). Some 79% of physicians reduce the dose of antihypertensive drugs once a normal blood pressure has been reached.

Physicians seem to have a rather low opinion of the value of health education through the mass media (Table 9). Still, most feel that public information lends support to the health profession's endeavours.

Where do physicians obtain information on hypertension control? Virtually all say they derive information from medical journals (Table 9). Two thirds each refer to continuing education programmes and information from the pharmaceutical industry. Neither WHO nor ISH are mentioned as an information source of any importance.

Table 3. Physician inquiry, Ashkelon: reported practices in blood pressure measurement

Question	Answers	Number of physicians
Who measures blood pressure in your office?	Physician	7
	Nurse	5
	Physician or nurse	18
How is blood pressure measured?	Right arm	6
	Left arm	8
	Both	16
	Sitting	22
	Lying	15
	Standing	6
What interval do you leave between measurements?	10.7 min (mean)	30
Which device do you use?	Mercury sphygmomanometer	30
How often do you standardize the device?	Yearly	15
	Every two years	3
	Less	12
Which Korotkoff sound do you use?	IV	17
	V	13
Do you record blood pressure values to the nearest 10 mmHg, 5 mmHg or 2 mmHg?	10 mmHg	7
	5 mmHg	18
	2 mmHg	5
Do you think self-measurement is useful?	No	1
	Yes	29
When did you last check your own blood pressure?	Last month	5
	Last year	25

Table 4. Physician inquiry, Ashkelon: information about physicians' practices

Question	Answers	Number of physicians
How many patients did you see last year?	1924 (mean)	30
How many hypertensive patients did you see last year?	112 (mean)	30
Do you keep a register of hypertensive patients?	No	1
	Yes	29
Do you use a reminder system for hypertensive patients?	No	8
	Yes	22
Do you actively invite your hypertensive patients for control?	No	3
	Yes	27
Do you think a personal computer in your office could help you in setting up a reminder system for your hypertensive patients?	No	4
	Yes	26

Table 5. Physician inquiry, Ashkelon: blood pressure levels physicians use to define hypertension

Blood pressure (mmHg)	Number (%) of physicians who define various blood pressure levels as hypertension in patients aged:		
	< 35 years	35 – 59 years	60 + years
Systolic			
140	21 (69)	4 (11)	–
150	7 (24)	10 (34)	1 (3)
160	2 (7)	16 (55)	29 (97)
Diastolic			
80	–	–	–
90	10 (34)	6 (21)	2 (7)
100	20 (66)	24 (79)	28 (93)

Table 6. Physician inquiry, Ashkelon: attitudes towards non-drug treatment as reflected by actions reported by physicians

Reported action	Physicians No.	(%)
Advise non-drug treatment		
weight reduction	30	(100)
sodium restriction	25	(83)
physical exercise	24	(80)
behavioural therapy	20	(65)
stopping oral contraception	22	(72)
other	14	(48)
Inquire about other cardiovascular disease risk factors		
smoking	30	(100)
hyperlipidaemia	28	(93)
alcohol consumption	28	(93)

Table 7. Physician inquiry, Ashkelon: procedures performed in the clinical work-up of hypertensive patients

Procedure	Physicians No.	(%)
Body weight	30	(100)
Height	25	(82)
Urine analysis	27	(90)
Electrocardiogram	30	(100)
Serum potassium	30	(100)
Serum creatinine	30	(100)
Serum cholesterol	30	(100)
Serum uric acid	28	(93)
Post-load blood sugar	24	(79)
Chest X-ray	27	(90)
Eye-ground examination	29	(96)

Table 8. Physician inquiry, Ashkelon: first choice of drugs

Drug	Number of physicians
Beta-blockers	21
Diuretics	20
Calcium antagonists	17
Vasodilators	7
Rauwolfia	0
Others (including combinations)	28

Table 9. Physician inquiry, Ashkelon: physicians' general attitudes towards hypertension control

Question	Answers	Number of physicians
Do you think that the activities concerning hypertension control are sufficient:		
on television?	No	20
	Yes	10
on radio?	No	23
	Yes	7
in newspapers?	No	23
	Yes	7
Do you think that information on hypertension via the media supports physicians' treatment of hypertensive patients?	No	10
	Yes	20
Do you think that continuous medication has negative psychological effects on your hypertensive patients?	No	15
	Yes	15
Do you think side effects of antihypertensive drugs must be accepted or tolerated by the patients?	No	27
	Yes	3
How do you usually obtain information on hypertension and other cardiovascular risk factors?	Medical journals	28
	Continuing education programmes	21
	Textbooks	21
	Pharmaceutical industry information	19
	Television/radio/newspapers	2
	Leagues against hypertension	1
	WHO	2
	ISH	0
	National high blood pressure education programme	6

11

A COMMUNITY SURVEY IN MUNICH, GERMANY

U. Keil, A. Döring & J. Stieber

A community survey was carried out in 1980 – 1981 in a random population sample of men and women aged 30 – 69 years in the City of Munich.

Foreigners, amounting to about 17% of the Munich population, were excluded. Of the 1.3 million inhabitants of Munich in 1980, 524 328 fulfilled the criteria of the study population and, of this number, a random sample amounting to 3400 people was drawn in October 1980. A comparison of the demographic particulars of the sample with the total population shows that the sample reflects the characteristics of the population as a whole. Some 202 people were lost owing to mortality, migration, etc. Of the remaining 3198 people, 2216 (69.3%) participated in the study. The sample sizes by sex and age group, and their response rate, are given in Table 1.

The table shows a slightly lower participation rate among women than among men, which was lowest among the oldest women.

Table 1. Community survey, Munich: age and sex composition of random sample (of 3198 people) and response rate

Age (years)	Male		Female	
	No.	response rate (%)	No.	response rate (%)
30 – 39	302	70	298	70
40 – 49	326	72	319	69
50 – 59	232	74	315	67
60 – 69	182	71	242	62
Total	1042	72	1174	67

Results

The Hawksley Random Zero Sphygmomanometer was used to measure blood pressure, and the measurement took place after completion of an interview averaging about 30 minutes. The prevalence of hypertension (defined as systolic blood pressure above 160 mmHg and diastolic blood pressure above 95 mmHg, or treatment for hypertension) in the various age groups is seen in Table 2. The expected increasing prevalence with increasing age is seen especially among women.

The rate of awareness among the hypertensive people is seen in Table 3. Although the prevalence of hypertension was similar in the two sexes, more men had never been told that they were hypertensive; 15% of all the men and women in the sample screened had been told at some time that they had hypertension. A total of 135 men and 162 women who had normal blood pressure and were not being treated claimed they had been told at some time that they had hypertension.

Table 2. Community survey, Munich: prevalence of hypertension by age and sex

Age (years)	Prevalence of hypertension (%)	
	Male	Female
30 – 39	11	3
40 – 49	22	13
50 – 59	32	25
60 – 69	32	36
Total	23	19

Table 3. Community survey, Munich: awareness and treatment status on first examination

Awareness and treatment status	Male			Female			Total		
	No.	% of sample screened	% of hyper-tensives	No.	% of sample screened	% of hyper-tensives	No.	% of sample screened	% of hyper-tensives
Total sample screened	1042	100	–	1174	100	–	2216	100	–
Total found hypertensive	237	23	100	217	19	100	454	21	100
Never told	90	9	38	34	3	16	124	6	27
Told at some time	147	14	62	183	16	84	330	15	73
Treated now	88	8	37	133	11	61	221	10	49

12

A METHODOLOGICAL EXERCISE IN VERNIER, SWITZERLAND

E. Brenner & A. Rougemont

A methodological exercise was carried out by postgraduate students to assess the awareness of hypertension in the community of Vernier, near Geneva, Switzerland.

Vernier is a residential community, with a number of smaller industrial plants, on the outskirts of Geneva, Switzerland. It has a population of 28 000. The well known international character of the city of Geneva is reflected in the structure of the population of Vernier; nevertheless, the 42% of foreigners living in Vernier are mostly modest and medium income guest workers, rather than the wealthier international civil servants. Health care in Geneva, as in Switzerland in general, is based on private medicine, most inhabitants being covered by some type of health insurance scheme. The main canton hospital is run by the State of Geneva; it also functions as a teaching hospital.

A campaign of mass screening for hypertension took place in Geneva ten years before the present study. Blood pressure was measured in all subjects attending for mass radiography, covering most employed individuals. People found to have elevated blood pressure were referred to their physicians.

Objectives

The present project was an exercise for students of a one-year postgraduate course of community medicine and epidemiology at the University of Geneva. Most of the 32 students were physicians or nurses, while some belonged to various other health-related professions. Each year the students carry out a community-based project dealing with a problem of public health importance. In 1988, the problem was that of awareness of hypertension in a community.

The project thus had several objectives: didactic, methodological and epidemiological.

The didactic objective was to initiate the postgraduate students into the techniques of planning and executing a population-based survey.

The methodological objective was to apply the cluster survey method to a particular problem. This method has been used by WHO's Expanded Programme on Immunization (EPI) to evaluate immunization coverage.

The epidemiological objective was to assess awareness of blood pressure in the population of the study community, by determining the proportion of adults who had had their blood pressure measured during the three months and during the year before the study, and by ascertaining the level of awareness of hypertension in the population.

Methods

As reported earlier,[a] the adopted survey design called for 24 clusters with the selection of 10 individuals per cluster. Although formal statistical theory requires a minimum of 30 clusters in this type of survey, for practical reasons 24 clusters were deemed sufficient in this exercise. Clusters were selected according to the standard EPI method, whereby any one of the exhaustively enumerated subpopulation has a probability of being selected which is proportional to the size of its population. The basis for the sampling was a local civil defence census that had divided the community into neighbourhood "islands" of 50 – 1000 individuals. In each cluster, a starting household was selected at random, after which surveyors proceeded to the next nearest household.

Survey teams consisted of two course participants, one of whom was always a physician or a nurse. Visits were made after working hours, around the time of the evening meal, to maximize the likelihood of finding people at home. Local authorities (including those responsible for public health services), the police, the press, and local physicians had been notified in advance about the survey.

Each individual surveyed was asked about his/her age and origin, as well as how long it had been since his/her blood pressure had been taken, on what occasion and by whom, and whether he/she knew what the results had been. Blood pressure was measured using a standardized method. Survey questionnaires were tabulated using the public domain statistical software EPI INFO, initially developed by the Centers for Disease Control in the United States, and more recently with the collaboration of the WHO Global Programme on AIDS.

Results

A total of 248 people were surveyed. Although the primary purpose of the study was not to screen for undetected hypertension, a number of people were found to have blood pressure in the range that might require medical attention. Therefore, all those found to have systolic pressures exceeding 140 mmHg and/or diastolic pressures exceeding 90 mmHg were referred to their own physicians, with a letter explaining the circumstances in which blood pressure had been measured.

The results shown in Fig. 1 indicated that blood pressure had been measured in nearly three quarters of the sample population within the last year. This includes both those who had had their blood pressure examined within the previous 3 months (43%) and those who had had a check 3 – 12 months before (29%). The 95% confidence intervals around these estimates were calculated to be ± 7%.

Table 1 presents information on the circumstances in which blood pressure was measured. In

[a] INSTITUTE OF SOCIAL AND PREVENTIVE MEDICINE, UNIVERSITY OF GENEVA. Chronic disease surveys. Evaluation of hypertension screening in a Swiss community using the cluster survey methodology of the EPI. *Weekly epidemiological record*, **65**: 331 – 333 (1990).

Fig. 1. Hypertension screening, Vernier: time since last blood pressure measurement

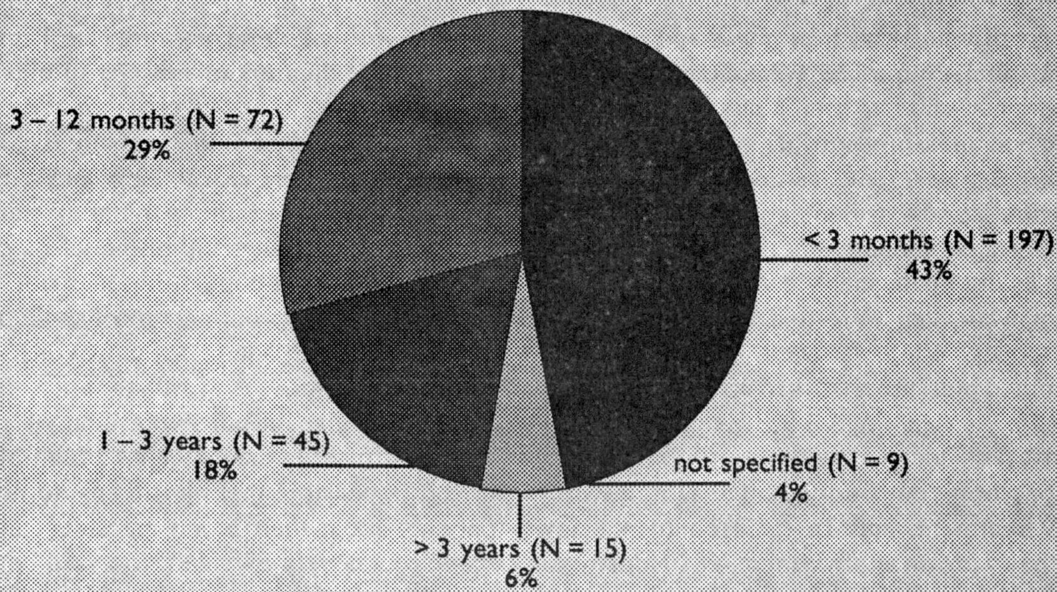

Source: Institute of Social and Preventive Medicine, University of Geneva, op. cit.

Table 1. Hypertension exercise, Vernier: circumstances in which blood pressure was measured

Circumstance	Respondents	
	No.	(%)
Self-measurement	6	(2)
Seeing doctor for hypertension	18	(7)
Seeing doctor for other reason	155	(63)
In hospital	27	(11)
Blood bank	9	(4)
In pharmacy	5	(2)
Other	22	(9)
No information	6	(2)
Total	248	(100)

most subjects (63%) blood pressure had been measured during a visit to a physician, for some reason other than hypertension. In some 11% of the subjects, blood pressure had been measured during a stay in hospital. Some 7% were actually hypertensive patients who had seen a physician because of high blood pressure. Further opportunities for blood pressure measurement were examinations of blood donors, self-measurement and the use of instruments located in pharmacies.

Table 2 sums up the interviewed subjects' recollections of what they were told about their blood pressure values. While 7% were aware of having elevated blood pressure, 10% had no recollection of the result.

Finally, 7% declared taking antihypertensive medication; only one individual was following non-drug treatment, and 16 (6%) could not say whether they were on antihypertensive treatment or not (Table 3).

Table 4 presents the blood pressure levels recorded by a team, trained in blood pressure measurement, in the homes of the surveyed subjects. Because of the modest sample size, the figures are not presented as frequency distributions of the actual values measured, but as normal versus elevated blood pressure findings.

Normal blood pressure was found in 74% of those surveyed. Of the 64 people with elevated values, 22 had an elevation of both systolic and diastolic pressure; in 30 people only systolic blood pressure and in 12 only diastolic were found above the cut-off points considered by WHO as normal.

A striking contrast appears when the figure of 64 people found to be above the normal range is compared with the 17 people who were aware of having elevated blood pressure (see Table 2). Thus, nearly three quarters of those with elevated blood pressure values were unaware of their condition, despite the fact that blood pressure *had* been measured within the last year in 72%, and within the last 3 years in 90% of the population sample. This finding indicates that a high rate of blood pressure measurement in a population does not necessarily equate with an appropriate rate of awareness nor, by implication, with adequate control of hypertension in the population.

It may also be an expression of physician's attitudes towards the concept of high blood pressure. It is possible that physicians do not tell their patients about their blood pressure values, unless they are severely elevated, to avoid causing them anxiety or labelling them. No information is available, however, on physicians' concepts in this area.

Conclusion

Elevated blood pressure values, i.e. at or above 140 mmHg and/or 90 mmHg, were found in 25% of the surveyed population. Most of the population had had their blood pressure measured in the relatively recent past, yet only 7% of the population were actually aware of having been told that they had elevated values. Blood pressure measurement by itself is no guarantee of adequate awareness or control.

Table 2. Hypertension exercise, Vernier: subjects' recollection of measurement results

Recollected results	Respondents No.	(%)
Blood pressure elevated	17	(7)
Blood pressure not elevated	186	(75)
Does not know	26	(10)
Measurement not made	3	(1)
No information	16	(7)
Total	248	(100)

Table 3. Hypertension exercise, Vernier: form of treatment received

Treatment	Respondents No.	(%)
Drugs	17	(7)
Other	1	(1)
None	199	(80)
Does not know	16	(6)
No information	15	(6)
Total	248	(100)

Table 4. Hypertension exercise, Vernier: blood pressure levels by age group

Blood pressure level		Age group (years) 18 – 30	31 – 40	41 – 50	51 – 60	61 +	All ages
Normal	No.	46	55	54	18	18	184
	% of blood pressure group	25	30	29	10	6	100
	% of age group	85	85	86	53	34	74
Systolic, over 140 mmHg	No.	6	3	2	5	14	30
	% of blood pressure group	20	10	7	17	47	100
	% of age group	11	5	3	15	44	12
Diastolic, over 90 mmHg	No.	2	3	2	5	0	12
	% of blood pressure group	17	25	17	42	0	100
	% of age group	4	5	3	15	0	5
Systolic, over 140 mmHg *and* diastolic, over 90 mmHg	No.	0	4	5	6	7	22
	% of blood pressure group	0	18	23	27	32	100
	% of age group	0	6	8	18	22	9
Total	No.	54	65	63	34	32	248
	% of age group	22	26	25	14	13	100

13

PHYSICIAN INQUIRY IN BOCHUM/DORTMUND, STUTTGART AND MUNICH, GERMANY

U. Keil, A. Spelsberg, S.K. Weiland, U. Härtel, H.-W. Hense & G. Pfaff

Inquiries into the knowledge, opinions and attitudes of physicians concerning hypertension were carried out in three samples of practising physicians in Bochum/Dortmund, Stuttgart and Munich.

Bochum and Dortmund are major cities of the Ruhr area in the north-western part of Germany. The two cities combined have a population of nearly one million people. Stuttgart, with a population of about half a million people, and Munich, with nearly 1.2 million inhabitants, are located in the south and the south-east of Germany, respectively.

Method

Since general practitioners and internists play a crucial role in the detection and management of most hypertensive patients, these two groups of physicians were targeted to participate in the study. A questionnaire was sent to every general practitioner or internist in the three study areas. The addresses were provided by the local physician organizations. In each area, the survey lasted ten weeks from the first mailing of the questionnaire to the end. The survey was completed in Bochum/Dortmund by the end of March 1988, in Stuttgart by the end of December 1986, and in Munich by the end of December 1985. Follow-up was performed by phone calls and two additional mailings. In Stuttgart, non-responders received up to four reminding letters but no phone calls.

The number of eligible physicians in each area and their response rates are shown in Table 1. The response rate was considerably lower in Munich (40%) than in the other two areas (around 70%).

Results

The reasons the physicians gave for measuring blood pressure in a patient are depicted in Table 2. The figures both for routine checking and for each patient group were lower in Munich than in the other two areas.

Table 1. Physician inquiry, Bochum/Dortmund, Stuttgart and Munich: study population

Study population	Physicians No.	Physicians response rate (%)
Bochum/Dortmund	442	71
Stuttgart	361	68
Munich	1251	40

Table 2. Physician inquiry, Bochum/Dortmund, Stuttgart and Munich: reasons for measuring blood pressure

Reason	Percentage of physicians in:		
	Bochum/ Dortmund	Stuttgart	Munich
Done routinely	68	77	71
Patient is known hypertensive	70	66	61
Done for every new patient	72	73	65
Hypertension is suspected	58	55	48
Hypotension is suspected	54	52	44

The role of nurses in blood pressure assessment is shown in Table 3. Between 67% and 79% of the general practitioners or internists reported involving nurses sometimes or more often in blood pressure measurements.

Table 4 gives the various positions in which blood pressure was taken. In general, the seated position was used.

As shown in Table 5, there was no general rule as to which arm was used in measuring blood pressure. Between 63% and 66% of physicians recorded Korotkoff sound V, and 14 – 21% used different cuff sizes. About 45% corrected the blood pressure values depending on the upper arm circumference.

The levels at which antihypertensive treatment was started are demonstrated in Table 6. The reported cut-off levels for drug treatment are very similar for the three areas.

Table 7 depicts the diagnostic procedures that physicians consider indispensable in the work-up of the newly detected hypertensive patient. No differences between the three study areas are observed. Urine analysis, serum creatinine determination and electrocardiogram recording were first-choice

Table 3. Physician inquiry, Bochum/Dortmund, Stuttgart and Munich: involvement of nurses in the blood pressure measurements

Frequency of involvement of nurses	Percentage of physicians in:		
	Bochum/ Dortmund	Stuttgart	Munich
Generally	7	3	5
Often	28	23	28
Sometimes	44	41	42
Never	20	33	24

Table 4. Physician inquiry, Bochum/Dortmund, Stuttgart and Munich: usual position in which blood pressure is taken

Position of patient	Percentage of physicians in:		
	Bochum/ Dortmund	Stuttgart	Munich
Supine	3	5	2
Seated	61	66	72
Standing	1	0	0
It varies	34	29	24

procedures. Determination of total cholesterol, serum potassium and fasting blood glucose as well as eye-ground examination were carried out less often.

The first choice drugs in antihypertensive treatment are shown in Table 8. Beta-blockers were clearly preferred for younger patients as were diuretics for the elderly, and there was a remarkably strong concordance between the three study areas.

Conclusion

The inquiries of three samples of general practitioners and internists about their knowledge, attitudes and management of hypertension revealed no major discrepancies between the different study areas. The results show that national and international guidelines for hypertension detection and management are not sufficiently adopted. Not all physicians monitored blood pressure regularly at each patient visit. This weakness might be improved by involving trained nurses and allied health professionals more often in the measurement process. Even more important is the fact that only 63 – 66% of the physicians correctly used Korotkoff sound phase V for diastolic blood pressure determination. Greater education is required to avoid the unjustified medical

Table 5. Physician inquiry, Bochum/Dortmund, Stuttgart and Munich: techniques of blood pressure measurement

Technique	Percentage of physicians in:		
	Bochum/ Dortmund	Stuttgart	Munich
Arm usually used			
Right arm	18	20	23
Left arm	14	15	16
It varies	47	45	37
Both arms	22	20	22
Phase V of Korotkoff sound used	63	66	66
Different cuff sizes applied	21	20	14
Blood pressure values corrected depending on circumference of the upper arm	48	44	46

treatment of patients misclassified as hypertensives by using Korotkoff sound phase IV. In contrast to this, drug therapy was initiated at higher values than recommended in the national and international guidelines. Under 20% of the German physicians would initiate drug therapy at diastolic values below 95 mmHg, while nearly all physicians (90%) claimed to start drug therapy at diastolic levels above 100 mmHg. Obviously, there is still some controversy among German physicians about the national and international guidelines. Continuing efforts are needed to further improve German practising physicians' knowledge, attitudes and management of one of the most important cardiovascular risk factors.

Table 6. Physician inquiry, Bochum/Dortmund, Stuttgart and Munich: level of sustained blood pressure values at which physicians always start drug treatment

Blood pressure (mmHg)	Cumulative percentage of physicians who always start drug treatment at various blood pressure levels, in:		
	Bochum/ Dortmund	Stuttgart	Munich
Systolic			
140 +	0	3	5
150 +	14	19	18
160 +	58	59	65
170 +	81	78	79
180 +	95	95	95
189 +	100	100	100
Diastolic			
90 +	13	13	15
95 +	45	44	46
100 +	91	90	90
105 +	95	95	94
109 +	100	100	100

Table 7. Physician inquiry, Bochum/Dortmund, Stuttgart and Munich: procedures always performed by physicians in the diagnostic work-up of hypertensive patients

Procedure	Percentage of physicians in:		
	Bochum/ Dortmund	Stuttgart	Munich
Urine analysis	86	92	85
Electrocardiogram	84	69	80
Serum potassium	57	61	52
Serum creatinine	87	87	84
Total cholesterol	74	71	68
High-density lipoprotein cholesterol	43	41	31
Serum uric acid	55	45	54
Fasting blood sugar	58	50	58
Chest X-ray	48	39	43
Eye-ground examination	53	51	55

Table 8. Physician inquiry, Bochum/Dortmund, Stuttgart and Munich: physicians' first choice drugs

First choice drug	Percentage of physicians in:		
	Bochum/ Dortmund	Stuttgart	Munich
Younger patients			
Beta-blockers	81	84	83
Calcium antagonists	6	4	4
ACE inhibitors	5	1	3
Diuretics	5	10	6
Vasodilators	2	0	1
Others	1	1	2
Elderly patients			
Diuretics	50	54	60
Calcium antagonists	29	24	18
ACE inhibitors	7	5	5
Vasodilators	6	4	8
Reserpine	5	8	4
Others	4	6	6

14

PHYSICIAN INQUIRY IN STUTTGART, GERMANY

A. Füller, U. Laaser, V. Schumann & M. Siegel

An inquiry was carried out in Stuttgart to assess discrepancies between attitudes and self-reported behaviour among physicians.

People's opinions and attitudes often do not tally with their behaviour and deeds. Physicians are obviously no exception to this rule. The present investigation shows that in the domain of hypertension, too, physicians often think one way and act another, particularly regarding non-drug treatment.

Method

A questionnaire based on the study protocol of the Hypertension Management Audit Project was mailed to all general practitioners, internists and gynaecologists in private practice in Stuttgart, a total of 480 in 1986. The main target group was the 358 general practitioners and internists, of whom 244 (68%) answered the questionnaire.

Results

Altogether, three quarters of the respondents affirmed that a healthier lifestyle is sufficient to reduce the blood pressure of hypertensive people (Table 1). The percentage of the general practitioners was somewhat higher than that of the internists. The

Table 1. Physician inquiry, Stuttgart: effect of lifestyle on blood pressure

Statement	Answers	General practitioners (N = 135) %	Internists (N = 105) %	Total (N = 240) %
In a large number of persons with hypertension, a healthier lifestyle will be sufficient to reduce their blood pressure	1. Agree completely	42	33	39
	2. Agree in part	37	39	38
	1 + 2	79	72	76

physicians thus implicitly indicated their willingness to refrain from using drugs for hypertension treatment and to prefer a change in lifestyle towards health promoting habits.

A sceptical attitude towards the usual prescription of drugs was also expressed by the agreement of nearly 50% that drugs are prescribed too soon to hypertensive patients (Table 2). This opinion implied an indirect criticism of the physicians' usual treatment behaviour.

A large proportion of the responding physicians (69%) favoured self-measurement of blood pressure; and agreement among internists was distinctly higher than that among their colleagues in general medicine (Table 3).

Important reasons for caution about the pharmacological therapy of mild hypertension were the widespread physical and emotional side effects of antihypertensive drugs. These effects were implicitly recognized by 58% of the physicians who agreed with the statement that permanent drug intake is a burden for many patients (Table 4).

To investigate not only their opinion of the value of non-drug measures, but also their reported implementation, the physicians were asked whether they told their patients about generally available offers such as lectures, courses or special health insurance rates to help improve their lifestyles. Most of the physicians gave such advice on nutrition, weight loss, sports and smoking (Table 5).

Table 2. Physician inquiry, Stuttgart: drug treatment for hypertensives

Statement	Answers	General practitioners (N = 135) %	Internists (N = 105) %	Total (N = 240) %
In general, drugs are prescribed too quickly to hypertensive patients	1. Agree completely	13	13	13
	2. Agree in part	33	40	36
	1 + 2	45	53	49

Table 3. Physician inquiry, Stuttgart: self-measurement of blood pressure

Statement	Answers	General practitioners (N = 135) %	Internists (N = 105) %	Total (N = 240) %
I consider the measuring of blood pressure by the hypertensive patient himself an effective means to increase the positive therapeutic results	1. Agree completely	25	34	29
	2. Agree in part	37	44	40
	1 + 2	62	78	69

Table 4. Physician inquiry, Stuttgart: the burden of permanent drug intake

Statement	Answers	General practitioners (N = 135) %	Internists (N = 105) %	Total (N = 240) %
Permanent drug intake is a burden for many patients	1. Agree completely	13	9	11
	2. Agree in part	47	46	47
	1 + 2	60	54	58

Table 5. Physician inquiry, Stuttgart: advice about improved lifestyles

	Answers	General practitioners and internists (N = 242) %
Do you inform your hypertensive patients about generally available offers (such as courses, lectures in adult evening classes, health insurance companies and the like) to improve health?	Relaxation	47
	Nutrition	88
	Weight	94
	Smoking	87
	Sports	76
	Others	7

Nearly 90% of the physicians treated mild hypertension exclusively with drugs (Table 6). This practice clearly goes against the recommendations of organizations such as WHO and WHL and against the physicians' own opinions about the relevance of non-drug treatment.

Nevertheless, some physicians (38%) did, at least sometimes, discontinue drug prescription after normalization of the patient's blood pressure, while 90% of the physicians said that, at least in some cases, they would reduce the drug dosage (Table 7).

The willingness of patients to adopt non-drug measures to reduce blood pressure was considered rather negatively (Table 8). In view of such an assessment, it is not surprising that more than 50% of the physicians were prepared to ignore the side effects of drugs (Table 9).

The possible influence of the pharmaceutical industry on doctors was investigated by a question about the source of information on hypertension. Of the physicians who were informed about hypertension largely by representatives of the pharmaceutical industry, 47% treated patients with diastolic blood pressure values of 95 mmHg or less with drugs. Of those who were not informed by such representatives, only 34% did so (Table 10).

Conclusion

The physicians implicitly expressed the conviction that they acted in accordance with the principle of the non-drug treatment of hypertension in their everyday practice. The opinions indicated overall that the primary health care physicians were oriented to health maintenance and health promotion without drugs. On the other hand, according to a health survey carried out in Stuttgart in 1985, more than three quarters of those interviewed never received advice about nutrition, and more than two thirds never received recommendations about sports or smoking. This finding indicates that health counselling may be more an ideal than a practice. Only 14% of the hypertensive patients were not treated with drugs, although 85% were mild hypertensives. The results suggest that hypertensive patients may be overmedicated by their physicians.

The following factors may explain these discrepancies:

- contradictions between an ideal self-image and everyday behaviour;
- factors in the health care system that favour drug prescription;
- the demands and preferences of patients;
- some influences of the pharmaceutical industry; and
- a lack of competence in health counselling techniques.

Table 6. Physician inquiry, Stuttgart: when drug treatment is necessary

Question	Answers	General practitioners (N = 132) %	Internists (N = 104) %	Total (N = 236) %
At what diastolic blood pressure values do you consider treatment necessary? (No range of systolic blood pressure given)	Diastolic blood pressure (mmHg)			
	< 90	1	1	1
	90 – 94	16	8	12
	90 – 100	90	89	89

Table 7. Physician inquiry, Stuttgart: changes in drug treatment after normalization

Question	Answers	General practitioners (N = 135) %	Internists (N = 105) %	Total (N = 240) %
Do you interrupt or discontinue drug prescription after normalization of a patient's blood pressure?	Never	12	18	15
	Seldom, in part	40	51	45
	Sometimes	36	26	32
	Often	7	4	6

Table 8. Physician inquiry, Stuttgart: patients' preferred treatment

Statement	Answers	General practitioners (N = 135) %	Internists (N = 105) %	Total (N = 240) %
Patients are more willing to take tablets regularly than to change their habits in any way	1. Agree completely	49	53	51
	2. Agree in part	39	36	38
	1 + 2	88	90	89

Table 9. Physician inquiry, Stuttgart: side effects of drugs

Statement	Answers	General practitioners (N = 135) %	Internists (N = 105) %	Total (N = 240) %
Patients have to accept side effects of drugs	1. Agree completely	8	21	14
	2. Agree in part	42	35	40
	1 + 2	50	56	53

Table 10. Physician inquiry, Stuttgart: drug prescription habits in relation to main source of information about treatment of hypertension

Question	Answers	Percentage of physicians whose main source of information was:	
		pharmaceutical industry (N = 182)	other sources (N = 94)
At what blood pressure level do you start drug treatment?	Diastolic blood pressure (mmHg)		
	< 95	14	13
	95 – 104	33	21
	> 105	88	86

15

PHYSICIAN INQUIRY IN CATALONIA, SPAIN

M. Torner i Soler

A physician inquiry was performed among all general practitioners working in the public primary health care system in Catalonia, Spain.

Method

A random sample of 427 physicians (18.1% of the whole study population) was obtained, and a self-administered questionnaire with a prepaid envelope was sent to all of them. The questionnaire was a slightly modified version of the questionnaire developed by the Hypertension Management Audit Project.

For those who did not respond to the first questionnaire, a second one was sent a month later and, if there was still no response, it was followed a month later by a telephone call. The letter was signed by the Health Minister of Catalonia and the president of the Advisory Council on Hypertension in Catalonia; the telephone call was made by a physician. The study was performed between November 1987 and January 1988.

Results

The response rate was 53% (226 valid questionnaires out of 427); excluding the administrative drop-out, i.e those who had retired or died, the response rate was 60%. Of the responses, 61% were obtained after the first letter, 21% after the second and 18% after the telephone call.

The techniques of blood pressure measurement are shown in Table 1. Measurements were usually taken by the physician. They were taken on both arms in only 30% of patients. The sitting position was used by 81% of physicians. To confirm the diagnosis, blood pressure was measured twice by 26% of physicians and three times or more by 72%. These figures seem fairly, but not fully, satisfactory. Mercury sphygmomanometers were used by 68%, and automatic devices by virtually none. The blood pressure devices were calibrated very seldom, and not at all by 66%. The Korotkoff sounds used were usually (78%) phase V, which is a reasonable figure. As many as 96% rounded off the blood pressure level at 5 or 10 mmHg.

The levels considered as a definition of hypertension, as a criterion for treatment, and as a sign of acceptably controlled hypertension are given in Tables 2 and 3, for both systolic and diastolic blood

Table 1. Physician inquiry, Catalonia: reported practices in blood pressure measurement

Reported practices	Percentage of physicians
Measurement taken:	
by physician	75
by nurse	16
Measurement taken:	
on right arm	23
on left arm	16
on both arms	30
on different arms	30
Routine measurement:	
in sitting position	81
in supine position	7
in various positions	12
To confirm diagnosis, blood pressure measured:	
only once	2
twice	26
three times or more	72
Device used	
mercury	68
aneroid	30
automatic	< 1
Device standardized:	
once a year	23
less often	1
never	66
Sounds used	
Korotkoff V	78
Korotkoff IV	16

Reported practices	Percentage of physicians
Values rounded off:	
at 10 mmHg	26
at 5 mmHg	70
at 2 mmHg	4
Physician's own blood pressure checked during last year	70

Table 2. Physician inquiry, Catalonia: meaning of various systolic blood pressure levels

Systolic blood pressure (mmHg)	Percentage of physicians who consider various blood pressure levels as:		
	normal (N = 221)	needing treatment (N = 212)	a sign of controlled hypertension (N = 210)
< 140	4	0	3
140 – 149	20	1	26
150 – 159	40	13	34
160 – 169	35	54	34
170 – 179	1	22	2
≥ 180	1	9	1

Table 3. Physician inquiry, Catalonia: meaning of various diastolic blood pressure levels

Diastolic blood pressure (mmHg)	Percentage of physicians who consider various blood pressure levels as:		
	normal (N = 224)	needing treatment (N = 226)	a sign of controlled hypertension (N = 219)
< 90	17	1	25
90 – 94	54	19	50
95 – 99	25	31	19
100 – 104	4	42	6
≥ 105	0	8	0

pressures. In general, blood pressure treatment was felt necessary in the range 160 – 169 mmHg systolic and 95 – 104 mmHg diastolic.

Some kind of registration of hypertensive patients was used by 95% of physicians, and 31% used a special register for hypertensives.

Table 4 presents the clinical work-up applied to patients with hypertension. Determinations of total cholesterol, blood sugar, serum creatinine, serum uric acid, body weight and urine analysis achieved the highest priorities (more than 65%) followed by eye-ground examination and electrocardiogram (60%) and serum potassium determination (49%).

Table 5 shows the percentages of physicians advising any type of non-drug treatment to their patients. High figures for body weight reduction (93%) and sodium restriction (98%) are found, but alcohol restriction (67%) and physical activity (63%) were also recommended quite often.

Table 6 gives the first, second and third drug choices for antihypertensive treatment in patients aged 25 – 60 years of age. Diuretics were given as a first choice by 78% of physicians, with all other drugs coming below 5%. In general, beta-blockers were the favourite second and third choice, followed by ACE inhibitor drugs, sympathicolytics and again diuretics.

Physicians' management of patients in whom the expected reduction in blood pressure is not achieved is seen from Table 7: 57% of physicians add another drug, 14% increase the dosage, and 14% change the drug.

Table 8 shows that 61% try lowering the dosage if the patient's blood pressure is reduced to an acceptable level.

Table 4. Physician inquiry, Catalonia: procedures performed in the clinical work-up of hypertensive patients by 221 physicians

Procedure	Percentage of physicians
Body weight	67
Height	38
Urine analysis	66
Electrocardiogram	60
Serum potassium	49
Serum creatinine	80
Total cholesterol	85
Serum uric acid	69
Blood sugar	81
Chest X-ray	40
Eye-ground examination	60

Table 5. Physician inquiry, Catalonia:
non-drug treatment
advised by 223 physicians

Treatment advised	Percentage of physicians
Body weight reduction	93
Sodium restriction	98
Physical activity	63
Alcohol restriction	67

Table 6. Physician inquiry, Catalonia:
221 physicians' first choice drug or second and third choice drug
in combination therapy for patients aged 25 – 60 years

Drug	Percentage of physicians who use various drugs:		
	as first choice	as second choice	as third choice
Diuretics	78	12	18
ACE inhibitors	5	15	13
Sympathicolytics	4	12	14
Beta-blockers	3	30	36
Calcium antagonists	3	11	8
Diuretics + beta-blockers	2	12	8
Diuretics + reserpine	5	7	0
Vasodilators	–	–	2

Table 7. Physician inquiry, Catalonia: therapeutic plan of 155 physicians if blood pressure reduction is not achieved

Action	Percentage of physicians
Add another drug	57
Increase dosage	14
Change drug	14
Indifferent	14
No answer	3

Table 8. Physician inquiry, Catalonia: control scheme of 203 physicians if blood pressure reduction is achieved

Action	Percentage of physicians
Reduce dosage	61
No changes	38
Remove drugs	1
No answer	1

16

DRUG UTILIZATION STUDY IN HUNGARY

F. Endrényi, B. Bella, E. Rab, E. Török & J. Duba

The utilization of drugs to treat hypertension was studied in Hungary through prescriptions issued between 1986 and 1989.

Drug utilization studies, when based on representative samples, may yield quantitative information on the prescribing habits of physicians. This information may be used to influence the medical profession to adjust its prescribing to up-to-date standards. Since hypertension is in practice mainly treated by drugs, drug utilization studies are an important component of the assessment of the quality of care given in hypertension.

Methods

Outpatient drug prescriptions throughout Hungary were analysed for the period 1986 – 1989, taking 1986 as the baseline. The ATC classification recommended by WHO's Drug Utilization Research Group was used, as indicated in the protocol (Annex 1). Drug quantities were expressed in defined daily doses per 1000 inhabitants per day (DDD/1000 inhabitants/day) according to the schedule published by the Nordic Council on Medicines *(1,2)*.

Since arterial hypertension is preponderantly treated in outpatient departments, inpatient drug consumption was not taken into account. Countrywide data were derived from the numbers of packages delivered to public pharmacies by Hungaropharma, the central drug supply agency in Hungary. Information on the local consumption of drugs dispensed in four communities (two of them also studied by the Hungarian audit project) was obtained from the local pharmacies. Population sizes were given by the National Office of Population Statistics.

Results

The results are given in Tables 1 – 8.

Centrally acting antiadrenergic agents (C 02 A) (Table 1). Although the countrywide utilization of reserpine has decreased by 65% since 1986, it increased during the same period by 60% in the community of Leninváros. This increase may be due to the arrival in this community of a physician with outdated prescribing habits. Methyldopa utilization has decreased countrywide by 37%. The most important change in this group occurred in the

Table 1. Drug utilization study, Hungary:
use of centrally acting antiadrenergic agents (C 02 A) in Hungary, 1986 – 1989

Drug (ATC code)	Community	Drug utilization (DDD/1000 inhabitants/day)				
		1986	1987	1988	1989	Percentage change 1986 – 1989
Reserpine (C 02 AA 02)	Mosonmagyaróvár	0.325	0.254	0.120	0.001	−99.70
	Paks	0.590	0.346	0.247	0.084	−85.77
	Nagymágócs	0.282	0.166	0.045	–	
	Leninváros	0.626	0.509	0.673	1.001	+59.9
	Outpatients in Hungary	0.778	0.587	0.479	0.272	−65.03
Methyldopa (C 02 AB 01)	Mosonmagyaróvár	6.309	4.838	3.626	2.449	−61.19
	Paks	14.645	13.076	13.229	8.688	−40.68
	Nagymágócs	12.460	18.046	21.109	22.066	+77.09
	Leninváros	5.823	4.748	4.317	2.733	−53.07
	Outpatients in Hungary	11.912	11.119	10.865	7.464	−37.34
Guanfacine (C 02 AC 02)	Mosonmagyaróvár	0.614	3.458	6.999	9.145	+1389.41
	Paks	0.155	1.091	3.340	3.327	+2046.45
	Nagymágócs	–	0.351	2.630	6.015	+1613.67
	Leninváros	0.360	1.252	1.900	2.382	+561.66
	Outpatients in Hungary	0.415	1.245	2.387	2.978	+617.59

utilization of guanfacine, which increased more than six times.

Drugs with peripheral action (C 02 C) (Table 2). Purchases of prazosin increased by 120% between 1986 and 1988. This may have been associated with the fact that an important rise in drug prices was anticipated. Sales figures thus include an accumulation of stocks, not necessarily increased consumption. (The price of this preparation has indeed tripled.) Debrisoquine utilization steadily decreased during the observation period. Preparations containing guanethidine and guanazodine have been deleted from the list of registered drugs, and accordingly disappeared from the drug scene in 1989.

Agents acting on arteriolar smooth muscle cells (C 02 D) (Table 3). Dihydralazine does not have an important place in this group (only 8%), but its utilization increased by 8.5% from 1986 to 1989. Verapamil utilization has increased most dynamically in this group, but still does not seem to have reached the level it deserves. Nifedipine utilization increased by 56% between 1986 and 1989. This is the most frequently prescribed drug in hypotensive therapy; it seems that in 1989 its utilization was reaching a plateau. Fendiline utilization is very low: 0.6 DDD/1000 inhabitants/day in 1989, a decrease of 44% since 1986. Nitrendipine was registered in Hungary only in 1989; though growing fast, its utilization is still several orders of magnitude below that of nifedipine, and seems to vary greatly in different regions of the country. The utilization of calcium antagonists overall shows an

Table 2. Drug utilization study, Hungary: use of peripherally acting antiadrenergic agents (C 02 C) in Hungary, 1986 – 1989

Drug (ATC code)	Community	Drug utilization (DDD/1000 inhabitants/day)				
		1986	1987	1988	1989	Percentage change 1986 – 1989
Prazosin (C 02 CA 01)	Mosonmagyaróvár	2.635	3.684	3.858	3.444	+ 30.70
	Paks	3.834	6.992	9.764	8.409	+ 119.32
	Nagymágócs	1.351	1.492	2.829	5.232	+ 287.26
	Leninváros	4.066	5.133	6.607	5.536	+ 36.15
	Outpatients in Hungary	3.643	6.083	8.024	7.438	+ 104.17
Guanethidine (C 02 CC 02)	Mosonmagyaróvár	0.008	0.042	–	–	
	Paks	0.013	0.011	0.012	–	
	Nagymágócs	0.613	0.462	0.141	–	
	Leninváros	0.073	0.056	–	–	
	Outpatients in Hungary	0.073	0.056	0.005	–	
Debrisoquine (C 02 CC 04)	Mosonmagyaróvár	0.287	0.304	0.066	0.092	– 67.95
	Paks	0.502	0.691	0.562	0.150	– 70.12
	Nagymágócs	0.557	0.151	0.076	0.038	– 93.17
	Leninváros	3.795	3.838	3.400	2.981	– 21.45
	Outpatients in Hungary	1.027	0.794	0.698	0.459	– 55.30
Guanazodine (C 02 CC 06)	Mosonmagyaróvár	–	0.016	–	–	
	Paks	0.049	0.061	0.027	–	
	Nagymágócs	–	–	–	–	
	Leninváros	–	0.011	–	–	
	Outpatients in Hungary	0.030	0.020	0.015	0.004	– 86.66

increasing trend: from 17.1 DDD/1000 inhabitants/day in 1986 to 26.0 DDD/1000 inhabitants/day in 1989. The 1988 figure of 27.8 is probably due to over-purchasing because of the expected rise in prices.

The utilization of fixed combinations of centrally acting antiadrenergic agents (essentially reserpine) and diuretics (Table 4) amounted in 1986 to 3.4 DDD/1000 inhabitants/day. By 1989, their use had decreased by 50%, as an expression of the modernization of drug therapy.

Agents acting on the *renin-angiotensin system (C 02 E)* (essentially captopril) are gaining in importance, as shown by a 750% increase during the observation period (Table 5). Their place in therapy is still modest, however, with 1.4 DDD/1000 inhabitants/day.

Diuretics (C 03) (Table 6). The most used diuretic is clopamide (13.6 DDD/1000 inhabitants/day), followed by furosemide (8.6 DDD/1000 inhabitants/day), chlorthalidone (3.7 DDD/1000 inhabitants/day) and spironolactone (3.0 DDD/1000 inhabitants/day).

Table 3. Drug utilization study, Hungary: use of agents acting on arteriolar smooth muscle (C 02 D) in Hungary, 1986 – 1989

Drug (ATC code)	Community	Drug utilization (DDD/1000 inhabitants/day)				
		1986	1987	1988	1989	Percentage change 1986 – 1989
Dihydralazine (C 02 DB 01)	Mosonmagyaróvár	4.161	4.279	3.826	2.858	– 31.32
	Paks	0.793	1.162	1.025	0.513	– 35.31
	Nagymágócs	0.413	0.563	0.488	0.706	+ 70.94
	Leninváros	0.680	0.758	0.669	0.481	– 29.27
	Outpatients in Hungary	2.179	2.479	2.752	2.357	+ 8.51
Verapamil (C 02 DE 01)	Mosonmagyaróvár			–	0.171	
	Paks			0.036	0.974	
	Nagymágócs	–	–	–	0.121	
	Leninváros			0.015	0.271	
	Outpatients in Hungary	0.147	0.199	0.199	0.454	+ 208.84
Nifedipine (C 02 DE 02)	Mosonmagyaróvár	30.628	36.556	51.003	40.894	+ 33.51
	Paks	14.658	16.128	17.421	21.522	+ 46.82
	Nagymágócs	17.441	12.689	9.582	32.554	+ 86.65
	Leninváros	9.664	15.095	14.732	22.563	+ 133.47
	Outpatients in Hungary	15.743	17.234	26.344	24.567	+ 56.05
Fendiline (C 02 DE 08)	Mosonmagyaróvár	1.004	0.842	0.975	0.453	– 54.89
	Paks	0.574	0.777	1.063	0.506	– 11.85
	Nagymágócs	0.581	0.427	1.487	1.312	+ 125.81
	Leninváros	0.936	0.813	0.730	0.324	– 65.39
	Outpatients in Hungary	1.192	1.035	1.135	0.666	– 44.12
Nitrendipine (C 02 DE 09)	Mosonmagyaróvár	–	–	–	0.063	
	Paks	–	–	–	0.202	
	Nagymágócs	–	–	–		
	Leninváros	–	–	–	0.114	
	Outpatients in Hungary	–	–	0.077	0.293	
All calcium antagonists (C 02 DE)	Mosonmagyaróvár	31.632	37.398	51.978	41.581	+ 31.45
	Paks	15.232	16.905	18.520	22.704	+ 34.30
	Nagymágócs	18.435	13.679	11.557	34.693	+ 88.19
	Leninváros	10.800	15.908	15.462	23.372	+ 116.40
	Outpatients in Hungary	17.082	18.488	27.755	25.980	+ 52.08

Table 4. Drug utilization study, Hungary: use of centrally acting antiadrenergic agents and diuretics in combination (C 02 L) in Hungary, 1986 – 1989

Drug (ATC code)	Community	Drug utilization (DDD/1000 inhabitants/day)				
		1986	1987	1988	1989	Percentage change 1986 – 1989
Reserpine + diuretics (C 02 LA 01)	Mosonmagyaróvár	6.682	6.232	4.931	3.844	– 42.48
	Paks	3.409	3.635	3.762	1.403	– 58.85
	Nagymágócs	1.977	2.076	1.308	0.768	– 61.15
	Leninváros	2.513	2.702	2.724	1.952	– 22.33
	Outpatients in Hungary	3.409	3.004	2.728	1.710	– 49.83

Table 5. Drug utilization study, Hungary: use of agents acting on the renin-angiotensin system (C 02 E) in Hungary, 1986 – 1989

Drug (ATC code)	Community	Drug utilization (DDD/1000 inhabitants/day)				
		1986	1987	1988	1989	Percentage change 1986 – 1989
Captopril (C 02 EA 01)	Mosonmagyaróvár	0.137	0.175	0.546	1.283	+ 836.49
	Paks	0.048	0.036	0.274	0.705	+ 1368.75
	Nagymágócs	–	0.082	0.090	0.852	+ 939.02
	Leninváros	0.116	0.419	0.329	0.319	+ 175.00
	Outpatients in Hungary	0.169	0.277	0.737	1.437	+ 750.29

Furosemide shows the greatest increase (34.3%). There was apparently a slight over-purchasing of diuretics in 1988, though the prices in this group rose only slightly.

Beta-blockers (C 07) (Table 7). Countrywide data indicate that this group is the third choice after antihypertensives (C 02) and diuretics (C 03). This sequence has not changed despite the rise in prices in 1988. Compounds and combinations within this group are used in the following order:

1. pindolol + clopamide
2. metoprolol
3. oxprenolol
4. pindolol
5. propranolol
6. chloranolol.

The use of fixed combinations thus leads, with 9.6 DDD/1000 inhabitants/day.

In summary (Table 8), the use of nonselective beta-blockers is greater than that of the selective ones (essentially metoprolol). In 1986, the use of nonselective beta-blockers amounted to 10.1 DDD/1000 inhabitants/day, as compared with 4.2 DDD/1000 inhabitants/day for selective beta-blockers.

Table 6. Drug utilization study, Hungary: use of diuretics (C 03) in Hungary, 1986 – 1989

Drug (ATC code)	Community	Drug utilization (DDD/1000 inhabitants/day)				
		1986	1987	1988	1989	Percentage change 1986 – 1989
Hydroclorothiazide (C 03 AA 03)	Mosonmagyaróvár	0.967	0.757	0.743	0.462	– 52.23
	Paks	0.867	1.080	1.081	0.751	– 13.38
	Nagymágócs	6.160	6.634	6.484	6.333	+ 2.80
	Leninváros	1.131	0.847	0.615	0.392	– 65.35
	Outpatients in Hungary	1.781	1.568	1.381	1.237	– 26.41
Chlorothiazide (C 03 AA 04)	Mosonmagyaróvár	0.003	–	–	–	
	Paks	–	–	–	–	
	Nagymágócs	–	–	–	–	
	Leninváros	0.008	–	–	–	
	Outpatients in Hungary	0.014	0.003	–	–	
Clopamide (plain) (C 03 BA 03)	Mosonmagyaróvár	16.231	17.945	20.880	18.626	+ 14.75
	Paks	11.875	11.924	13.391	8.708	– 26.67
	Nagymágócs	7.170	8.187	11.303	13.521	+ 88.57
	Leninváros	7.548	9.482	7.482	8.737	+ 15.75
	Outpatients in Hungary	12.574	12.886	15.419	13.650	+ 8.55
Chlortalidone (C 03 BA 04)	Mosonmagyaróvár	0.942	0.863	1.081	1.399	+ 48.51
	Paks	3.376	3.410	3.385	2.226	– 34.07
	Nagymágócs	0.312	0.316	0.295	1.147	+ 267.62
	Leninváros	8.399	5.277	5.016	5.005	– 40.41
	Outpatients in Hungary	7.228	4.114	4.875	3.751	– 40.58
Furosemide (C 03 CA 01)	Mosonmagyaróvár	8.232	8.211	9.791	9.276	+ 12.68
	Paks	6.700	8.610	7.944	5.667	– 15.42
	Nagymágócs	7.140	8.564	6.975	9.346	+ 30.89
	Leninváros	2.933	3.670	3.780	4.025	+ 37.23
	Outpatients in Hungary	6.403	7.222	8.013	8.598	+ 34.28
Etacrynic acid (C 03 CC 01)	Mosonmagyaróvár	0.435	0.305	0.537	0.561	+ 28.96
	Paks	0.362	0.343	0.400	0.422	+ 16.57
	Nagymágócs	0.178	0.151	–	0.168	– 5.61
	Leninváros	0.125	0.142	0.347	0.271	+ 116.80
	Outpatients in Hungary	0.369	0.385	0.451	0.384	+ 4.06

Table 6 (contd)

Drug (ATC code)	Community	Drug utilization (DDD/1000 inhabitants/day)				
		1986	1987	1988	1989	Percentage change 1986 – 1989
Spironolactone (C 03 DA 01)	Mosonmagyaróvár	5.272	5.965	6.420	5.839	+ 10.75
	Paks	2.496	2.883	3.640	2.438	– 2.33
	Nagymágócs	3.001	2.716	2.202	2.506	– 16.49
	Leninváros	0.750	1.050	0.928	0.869	+ 15.86
	Outpatients in Hungary	3.125	3.181	3.428	3.011	– 3.64
All diuretics (plain) (C 03)	Mosonmagyaróvár	32.082	34.046	39.452	36.163	+ 12.72
	Paks	25.676	28.250	29.841	20.212	– 21.29
	Nagymágócs	23.961	26.568	27.259	33.021	+ 37.81
	Leninváros	20.894	20.468	18.168	19.249	– 7.88
	Outpatients in Hungary	31.494	29.359	33.567	30.631	– 2.74

With the increasing use of metoprolol, this difference had decreased by 1989 to 8.5 DDD/1000 inhabitants/day of nonselective beta-blockers versus 6.8 DDD/1000 inhabitants/day of selective beta-blockers. Overall, the use of antihypertensives, diuretics and beta-blockers increased by 13.28% between 1986 and 1989.

International Comparisons

The group of antihypertensives (C 02) is utilized in Hungary twice as much as in Finland or Sweden (Table 9). ACE inhibitors are used much less in Hungary, but are on the increase. Diuretics are also used much less than in Finland or Sweden *(3,4)* (Table 10). The overall use of beta-blockers does not differ much from that in Finland or Sweden; however, nonselective beta-blockers prevail in Hungary (by 3 : 1) while in Finland and Sweden the proportion is 2 : 1 in favour of selective beta-blockers (Table 11).

In the United States in 1989, calcium antagonists were the leading group (27%), followed by beta-blockers (23%) and ACE inhibitors (21%) *(5)*.

Conclusions

In summary, antihypertensives (C 02) are the most frequently prescribed group of drugs in the treatment of hypertension in Hungary. Within this group, in 1989, calcium antagonists were the most used drugs: accounting for 52% of the total use of 50.1 DDD/1000 inhabitants/day in this group. Diuretics (C 03) follow in second place with 30.6 DDD/1000 inhabitants/day, and beta-blockers (C 07) rank third with 15.3 DDD/1000 inhabitants/day. Prescriptions of antihypertensives, diuretics and beta-blockers together amount to 105 DDD/1000 inhabitants/day, meaning that virtually 1 in 10 inhabitants is being treated for hypertension. In 1988, over-purchasing occurred in all groups, due to the expected rise in prices; this was

Table 7. Drug utilization study, Hungary: use of beta-blockers (C 07) in Hungary, 1986 – 1989

Drug (ATC code)	Community	Drug utilization (DDD/1000 inhabitants/day)				
		1986	1987	1988	1989	Percentage change 1986 – 1989
Oxprenolol (C 07 AA 02)	Mosonmagyaróvár	4.126	4.031	3.690	3.102	– 24.82
	Paks	5.814	5.761	5.693	4.301	– 26.03
	Nagymágócs	5.277	5.394	5.467	6.773	+ 28.35
	Leninváros	9.988	11.082	10.549	7.868	– 21.23
	Outpatients in Hungary	4.177	4.242	4.177	3.605	– 13.69
Pindolol (C 07 AA 03)	Mosonmagyaróvár	2.859	3.522	4.214	4.065	+ 42.18
	Paks	2.321	2.316	2.168	1.267	– 45.41
	Nagymágócs	0.906	0.935	1.483	1.629	+ 79.80
	Leninváros	2.050	1.862	2.017	1.401	– 31.66
	Outpatients in Hungary	3.161	3.233	3.278	2.542	– 19.58
Propranolol (C 07 AA 05)	Mosonmagyaróvár	3.443	3.111	3.564	3.078	– 10.61
	Paks	0.821	1.395	1.132	1.039	+ 26.55
	Nagymágócs	3.118	3.534	4.294	5.086	+ 63.11
	Leninváros	1.080	1.088	1.486	1.179	+ 9.16
	Outpatients in Hungary	2.268	2.366	2.406	1.964	– 13.40
Cloranolol (C 07 AA 27)	Mosonmagyaróvár	1.137	0.688	0.506	0.438	– 61.48
	Paks	0.682	0.852	0.867	0.785	+ 15.10
	Nagymágócs	0.030	0.121	0.151	0.245	+ 716.66
	Leninváros	0.408	0.401	0.339	0.308	– 24.51
	Outpatients in Hungary	0.470	0.468	0.457	0.379	– 19.36
Metoprolol (C 07 AB 02)	Mosonmagyaróvár	6.497	6.482	7.660	7.778	+ 19.71
	Paks	2.046	3.359	5.541	4.441	+ 117.05
	Nagymágócs	0.645	1.228	1.308	1.522	+ 135.96
	Leninváros	3.854	5.517	5.143	9.493	+ 146.31
	Outpatients in Hungary	4.187	5.153	6.807	6.815	+ 62.76
All beta-blockers (plain) (C 07 A)	Mosonmagyaróvár	18.062	17.834	19.634	18.461	+ 2.20
	Paks	11.684	10.345	15.401	11.833	+ 1.27
	Nagymágócs	9.976	11.212	12.703	15.255	+ 52.91
	Leninváros	17.380	19.950	19.534	20.249	+ 16.50
	Outpatients in Hungary	14.263	15.462	17.125	15.305	+ 7.52

Table 7 (contd)

Drug (ATC code)	Community	Drug utilization (DDD/1000 inhabitants/day)				
		1986	1987	1988	1989	Percentage change 1986 – 1989
Pindolol + diuretics (C 07 CA 03)	Mosonmagyaróvár	20.230	25.821	29.801	26.893	+ 32.93
	Paks	11.194	11.396	15.237	12.029	+ 7.45
	Nagymágócs	0.935	2.005	3.223	8.092	+ 765.45
	Leninváros	12.345	15.433	18.106	15.252	+ 23.54
	Outpatients in Hungary	7.171	8.466	10.804	9.640	+ 34.43

followed by a general decrease in sales, with the notable exceptions of captopril, guanfacine, furosemide and metoprolol. In 1989, the most frequently used compounds were as follows:

1. nifedipine (24.6)
2. clopamide (plain) (13.6)
3. pindolol + diuretics (9.6)
4. furosemide (8.6)
5. methyldopa (7.4)
6. prazosin (7.4)
7. metoprolol (6.8)
8. oxprenolol (3.6 DDD/1000 inhabitants/day).

Prescribing habits in Hungary differ substantially from those in the Nordic countries and the United States.

References

1. *Guidelines for ATC classification.* Uppsala, Nordic Council on Medicines, 1990.
2. Endrényi, F. *A gyógyszerutilizáció gyakorlati kérdései* [Practical questions of drug utilization]. Budapest, Organization, Planning and Information Centre of the Ministry of Health, 1987.
3. *Suomen laaketilasto* [Finnish statistics on medicines]. Helsinki, Laakeing, 1989.
4. *Svensk lakemedelsstatistik 1988* [Swedish statistics on medicines, 1988]. Stockholm, Apoteksbolaget, 1989.
5. *European chemical news*, **54** (1417): 26 (1990).

Table 8. Drug utilization study, Hungary: summary of use of antihypertensives, diuretics and beta-blockers in Hungary, 1986 – 1989

Drug (ATC code)	Drug utilization (DDD/1000 inhabitants/day)			
	1986	1987	1988	1989
Antihypertensives (C 02)	*40.717*	*44.152*	*56.445*	*50.099*
Reserpine	0.778	0.587	0.479	0.272
Guanfacine	0.415	1.245	2.387	2.978
Methyldopa	11.912	11.119	10.865	7.464
Prazosin	3.643	6.083	8.024	7.438
Guanethidine, guanazodine	1.130	0.870	0.718	0.463
Dihydralazine	2.179	2.479	2.752	2.357
Captopril	0.169	0.277	0.737	1.437
Reserpine + diuretics	3.409	3.004	2.728	1.710
Calcium antagonists	17.082	18.488	27.755	25.980
Diuretics (C 03)	*31.494*	*29.359*	*33.567*	*30.631*
Thiazides (plain)	1.795	1.571	1.381	1.237
Sulfonamides (plain)	19.802	17.000	20.294	17.401
Furosemide and etacrynic acid	6.772	7.607	8.464	8.982
Potassium-sparing (spironolactone)	3.125	3.181	3.428	3.011
Beta-blockers (C 07)	*14.263*	*15.462*	*17.125*	*15.305*
Selective (metoprolol)	4.187	5.153	6.807	6.815
Nonselective	10.076	10.309	10.318	8.490
Beta-blockers + diuretics in combination (pindolol + clopamide)	*7.171*	*8.466*	*10.804*	*9.640*
Total	93.645	97.439	117.941	105.675

Table 9. Drug utilization study, Hungary: use of antihypertensives (C 02) in Finland, Sweden and Hungary

Drug group (ATC code)	Drug utilization (DDD/1000 inhabitants/day)								
	Finland			Sweden			Hungary		
	1986	1987	1988	1986	1987	1988	1986	1987	1988
Centrally acting antiadrenergic agents									
(C 02 A)	3.6	3.4	2.54	0.6	0.5	0.4	13.105	12.951	13.731
(Methyldopa)	(1.4)	(1.17)	(0.94)				(11.912)	(11.119)	(10.865)
C 02 L		1.77	1.47	< 0.1	< 0.1	< 0.1	3.409	3.004	2.728
Peripherally acting antiadrenergic agents									
(C 02 C)	7.2	7.01	6.00	1.4	1.2	1.1	5.943	6.953	8.742
Agents acting on arteriolar smooth muscle									
(C 02 D)	9.0	11.21	14.57	15.7	16.6	17.2	19.254	20.947	27.755
(Verapamil)	(4.2)	(4.62)	(4.84)				(0.147)	(0.199)	(0.199)
(Nifedipine)	(3.3)	(3.88)	(4.44)				(15.743)	(17.234)	(26.347)
Agents acting on renin-angiotensin system									
(C 02 E)	0.6	2.48	4.67	2.1	3.4	4.6	0.169	0.307	0.737
All antihypertensives									
(C 02)	20.4	25.87	29.25	19.9	21.8	23.4	41.88	44.162	56.444

Table 10. Drug utilization study, Hungary:
use of diuretics (C 03) in Finland, Sweden and Hungary

Drug group (ATC code)	Drug utilization (DDD/1000 inhabitants/day)								
	Finland			Sweden			Hungary		
	1986	1987	1988	1986	1987	1988	1986	1987	1988
Thiazides (C 03 A)	3.3	3.65	3.34	22.5	20.9	18.8	1.795	1.571	1.381
Sulfonamides (C 03 B)	1.6	1.32	1.08	3.1	2.7	2.3	19.802	17.000	20.294
Furosemide and etacrynic acid (C 03 C)	13.5	13.97	13.91	41.5	43.3	45.1	6.772	7.607	8.464
Potassium-sparing (C 03 D)	2.0	2.07	1.97	10.5	11.3	11.5	3.125	3.181	3.428
Diuretics in combination	43.9	43.93	42.82	12.3	12.7	12.4	3.586	4.233	5.402
All diuretics (C 03)	64.3	64.94	63.12	89.9	90.9	90.1	35.080	33.592	38.969

Table 11. Drug utilization study, Hungary:
use of beta-blockers (C 07) in Finland, Sweden and Hungary

Drug group (ATC code)	Drug utilization (DDD/1000 inhabitants/day)								
	Finland			Sweden			Hungary		
	1986	1987	1988	1986	1987	1988	1986	1987	1988
Selective (C 07 AA)	...	21.50	22.26	21.7	22.6	22.9	4.187	5.153	6.807
Non-selective and combinations with diuretics (C 07 AB)	...	11.77	11.04	11.8	11.2	10.3	17.247	18.775	21.122
All beta-blockers	33.2	33.27	33.30	33.5	33.8	33.2	21.434	23.928	27.929

17

DRUG UTILIZATION STUDY IN THE DISTRICT OF NOVI SAD

M. Stanulović, A. Sabo, V. Jakovljević & M. Planojević

The utilization of drugs to treat hypertension was studied in the District of Novi Sad, through drug prescriptions issued in 1985 and 1987.

Novi Sad is a town of 130 000 inhabitants; the district of Novi Sad includes some 200 000 inhabitants. The city is the administrative centre of the Province of Vojvodina, in the north-eastern part of the former Yugoslavia; the Provincial Parliament and Government, a university and a number of industrial and commercial enterprises are located in this city. The medical faculty of the university and the city health services have been actively involved for the past 15 years in various WHO programmes for the control and prevention of cardiovascular diseases, the main reason being the high and still increasing cardiovascular morbidity and mortality in the Province. The programmes include mass screening of the population, health education of the general public, continuing education of local physicians, and adjustments to the health services, aiming at an integrated programme to control the major noncommunicable diseases. The health services also participate in the WHO MONICA study, which includes screening a study sample of the population, yielding information on the prevalence of arterial hypertension among other things.

As in many other communities, hypertension is perceived as a major public health problem in Novi Sad; like elsewhere, however, little is known about the level and quality of the control of hypertension in the population. The assessment of drug prescription practices seemed to be a viable way of obtaining information on an important aspect of hypertension control: the utilization of antihypertensive drugs.

Methods

Data on drug use by the population aged 25 – 64 years were analysed for the years 1985 and 1987. For 1985, data were derived manually from a 10% sample of all prescriptions, processed by the pharmacies in the Novi Sad District during one week each in March, May, August and December.

For 1987, complete computerized information on all drugs prescribed during the whole year was available.

The prevalence of hypertension was already known from the survey of a 2% study sample of the population, aged 25 – 64 years, carried out in the context of the MONICA project. The sample included 1586 people. Blood pressure was measured twice by specially trained staff in health centres.

Results

A summary of the drug prescriptions for the population is given in Table 1. The total volume of hypertensive drug utilization in 1985 was 56.8 DDD/1000 inhabitants/day and, in 1987, 64.1. The most frequently prescribed drugs were combinations of diuretics, vasodilators and reserpine, and other hypotensives.

The prevalence of hypertension obviously depends on the cut-off points chosen, as shown in Table 2.

If hypertension is defined as persistent blood pressure values at or above 160/95 mmHg (the WHO criteria), a 7.5% prevalence is found in the population aged 25 – 64 years. If borderline values (above 150/85 mmHg) are added, the prevalence rises to 16.5%.

Discussion

Consumption of antihypertensive drugs varies widely from country to country *(1 – 3)*, as shown also in Chapters 16 and 18. A consumption of 64.1 DDD/1000 inhabitants/day in 1987, and even more so that of 56.8 DDD/1000 inhabitants/day in 1985, is considerably lower than that in a number of other populations. Nevertheless, the 1987 figure is in keeping with the prevalence of established hypertension found in the population of Novi Sad District, as shown in Table 2. The prevalence of 7.5% corresponds well with a consumption of 64.1 DDD/1000 inhabitants/day, considering that at least 10% of hypertensive patients should be manageable with non-drug treatment, without antihypertensive drugs.

Table 1. Drug utilization study, Novi Sad: drugs prescribed to the population aged 25 – 64 years in 1985 and 1987

Drug group	DDD/1000 inhabitants/day	
	1985	1987
Beta-blockers	7.4	5.0
Diuretics	11.0	7.5
Diuretics + sympathicolytics	1.4	0.6
Diuretics + vasodilators + reserpine	19.0	24.9
Calcium antagonists	8.2	5.8
Other[a]	9.8	20.3
Total	56.8	64.1

[a] Guanethidine, guanoxan, trimetaphan, dihydralazine, prazosin, diazoxide, sodium nitroprusside, indapamide.

Table 2. Drug utilization study, Novi Sad: prevalence of hypertension in a study sample of 1586 people

Study sample	Total	Borderline (150/85 mmHg)		Hypertensive (160/95 mmHg)		Borderline and hypertensive	
		No.	(%)	No.	(%)	No.	(%)
Males	795	73	(9)	53	(7)	126	(16)
Females	791	68	(9)	66	(8)	134	(17)
Both sexes	1586	141	(9)	119	(7.5)	260	(16.5)

At first sight the moderate or, in international comparisons, low consumption of antihypertensive drugs speaks in favour of a rational, appropriate drug utilization in the population. Such a conclusion presupposes, however, that the drugs are being used correctly on the individual level: that the right person takes the right medicament in the right dose. Obviously, this type of information cannot be derived from the present drug utilization study, but could be obtained in future from a more comprehensive implementation of the Hypertension Management Audit Project protocol (using the community and patient surveys).

Conclusion

Although the first impression is that of an adequate consumption of antihypertensive drugs in Novi Sad, the drug prescription study needs to be complemented with a more in-depth analysis of patient management. Although neither over- nor underconsumption of antihypertensive drugs seems to occur at the population level, this fact alone does not warrant a presumption of adequate drug utilization.

References

1. Jakovljević, V. et al. Prescribing of drugs for treatment of cardiovascular diseases in Novi Sad, Yugoslavia. *Physiologica pharmacologica acta*, **24**: 243 – 249 (1988).
2. Sabo, A. & Stanulović, M. Are we treating enough patients for hypertension? *International journal of clinical pharmacology, therapy and toxicology*, **26**: 194 – 198 (1988).
3. Stanulović, M. & Jakovljević, J. Extremes in drug utilization patterns. *Acta medica scandinavica* (Suppl.) (1984).

18

DRUG UTILIZATION STUDY IN SLOVENIA

P. Jezeršek & P. Dolenc

The utilization of drugs to treat hypertension was studied in Slovenia, through drug prescriptions issued in 1988.

In 1988, Slovenia had nearly 2 million inhabitants. The 40 – 69-year age group consisted of 652 450 people. Since, as shown in Chapter 6, the prevalence of hypertension in this group is close to 20%, an estimated 130 000 of these people were hypertensive. Data obtained in 1986 have shown that about 80% of hypertensives were on drug treatment.

The pharmacological classification of antihypertensive drugs used in this study distinguished six major groups:

- diuretics
- beta-blockers
- vasodilators
- calcium antagonists
- ACE inhibitors
- centrally acting antiadrenergic agents.

A group of fixed drug combinations should also be taken into account.

Computerized control of drug prescriptions was introduced in Slovenia in 1977. In 1988, 902 546 prescriptions for antihypertensive drugs were issued; this means an estimated average of seven prescriptions (or 14 packages of drugs) per hypertensive patient in that year. A single prescription can contain only the quantity of drugs sufficient for two months. Most antihypertensive prescriptions (94%) were administered to patients over 40 years of age.

The overall cost of antihypertensive drug treatment in Slovenia in 1988 amounted to US $4 199 109. Cost/benefit ratios can be estimated from data obtained by epidemiological studies of hypertension in Slovenia. As a result of drug treatment, only some 30% of hypertensives had achieved normal blood pressure values. Despite drug treatment, 68% of the hypertensives still had blood pressure values above the normal range.

All the major pharmacological groups of antihypertensive drugs are being used. Utilization has the following cost structure, computed from the expenditure on all antihypertensive drugs in 1988:

- calcium antagonists 31.7%
- fixed drug combinations 23.4%
- beta-blockers 14.8%
- ACE inhibitors 11.0%
- vasodilators 10.3%
- diuretics 6.1%
- centrally acting antiadrenergic agents 2.7%.

The cost of treatment with various antihypertensive drugs can vary considerably. If the cost of treatment with a frequently used fixed drug combination (Brinerdine),[a] is taken as 1.0 (the relative price of 1 DDD), the resulting average relative costs for other antihypertensive drug groups are as shown in column (a). Taking the cost of a standard diuretic for the basis of comparison, the average relative costs of the other drugs are as shown in column (b).

Drugs	(a)	(b)
Diuretics	0.9	1.0
Calcium antagonists	1.9	2.1
Beta-blockers	2.1	2.3
Centrally acting antiadrenergic agents	2.4	2.7
Vasodilators	2.6	2.9
ACE inhibitors	4.8	5.3

The utilization of antihypertensive drugs prescribed in Slovenia in 1988 is shown in Fig. 1. The largest column represents fixed drug combinations (31.5% of total DDDs of 189.7). The drug groups that follow are diuretic agents (26%), calcium antagonists (23%), beta-blockers (9.5%), vasodilators (5.4%), ACE inhibitors and centrally acting antiadrenergic drugs (1.5%). The WHO recommendation to start antihypertensive treatment with a single substance has obviously not been followed.

The most used diuretic agent is furosemide, followed by a combination of amiloride and hydrochlorothiazide (Moduretic) (Fig. 2). As the reason for prescribing a particular drug cannot be determined from the prescription, we believe that only a small proportion of loop diuretics is being used for the treatment of hypertension; loop diuretics are probably more often used in other diseases, such as congestive heart failure, liver cirrhosis, or the nephrotic syndrome.

Among the calcium antagonists (Fig. 3), a frequently used drug is verapamil. In Slovenia, however, this drug is not usually prescribed as an antihypertensive agent; it is more often used for the treatment of arrhythmias, paroxysmal tachycardias and similar disorders.

No particular beta-blocker is preferred in the treatment of hypertension (Fig. 4). The predominant beta-blocker tends to change from year to year. ACE inhibitors are only seldom prescribed, probably because of their high price.

The use of centrally acting adrenergic agents is historically conditioned. Methyldopa is still prescribed occasionally. Rauwolfia alkaloids are not available in monosubstance form, but are frequently used in combinations.

The drug most often prescribed in the group of fixed combinations is Brinerdine, followed by similar compound combinations (Fig. 5). The domination of this group in the consumption of antihypertensive drugs in Slovenia is surprising, when rational fixed drug combinations are available.

The use of Hydergin (Redergin) is unexpectedly high. Although the antihypertensive effects of this drug are in some doubt, the number of prescriptions is extensive. The probable explanation is that Hydergin is often prescribed as a geriatric medicine

[a] Brinerdine: clopamide 5.0 mg, reserpine 0.1 mg, dihydroergocristine 0.5 mg.

Fig. 1. Drug utilization study, Slovenia: consumption of antihypertensive drugs in the population aged 40 – 69 years

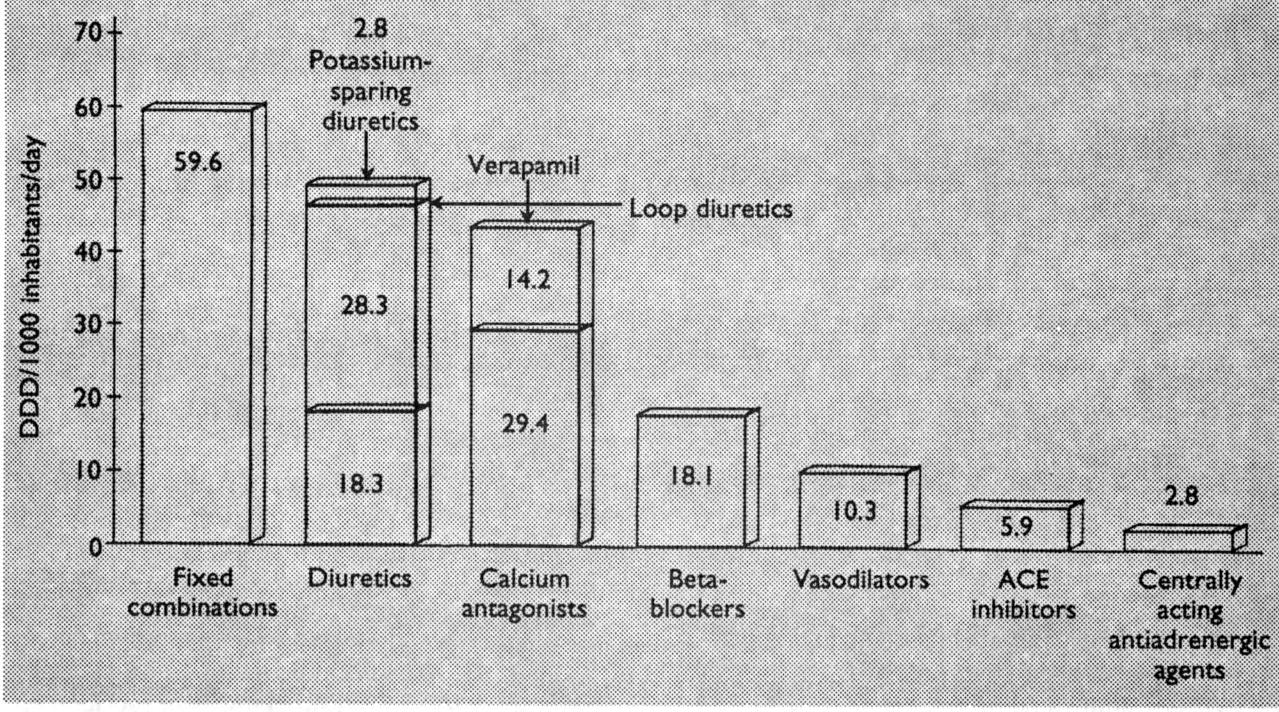

to improve cerebral perfusion. The total expenditure on Hydergin prescriptions in 1988 amounted to US $1 250 400 and is not included in the data analysis.

Price is also an important aspect of antihypertensive treatment and physicians are well aware of it. When deciding on the prescription, the physician has to consider the patient's personal characteristics, including his/her risk profile and likely compliance, as well as the properties, side effects and cost of the particular drug.

Our aim was to evaluate the dimensions and specificities of drug utilization in Slovenia. The prescribing of drugs is not a static phenomenon, but is subject to considerable variations. A comparison of the utilization of antihypertensive drugs between 1987 and 1988 has shown the following changes:

- reduction in usage of beta-blockers of about 5%;
- reduction in usage of fixed combinations of about 5%;
- reduction in usage of diuretics of about 45%;
- reduction in usage of centrally acting andiadrenergic agents of about 60%;
- increase in usage of vasodilators of about 10%;
- increase in usage of calcium antagonists of about 25%;

Fig. 2. Drug utilization study, Slovenia: a breakdown of the individual diuretics prescribed (in DDD/1000 inhabitants/day)

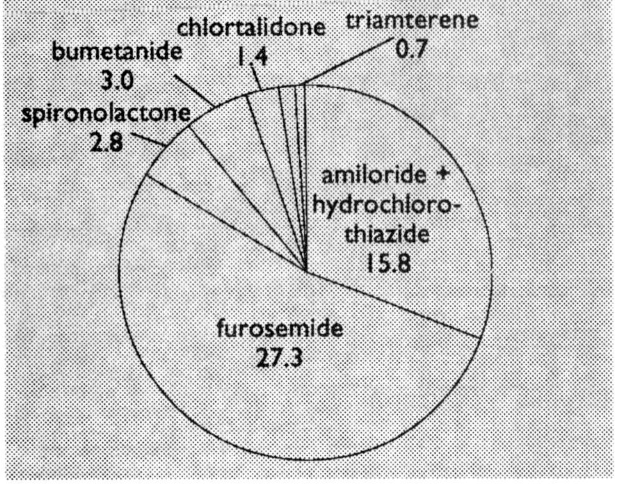

Fig. 3. Drug utilization study, Slovenia: a breakdown of the individual calcium antagonists prescribed (in DDD/1000 inhabitants/day)

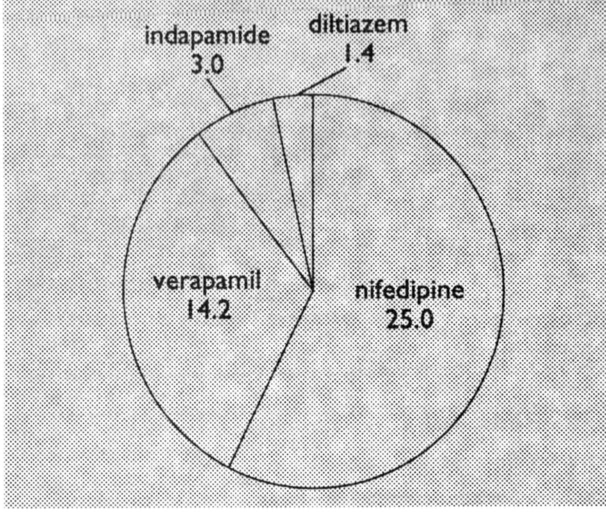

Fig. 4. Drug utilization study, Slovenia: a breakdown of the individual beta-blockers (in DDD/1000 inhabitants/day)

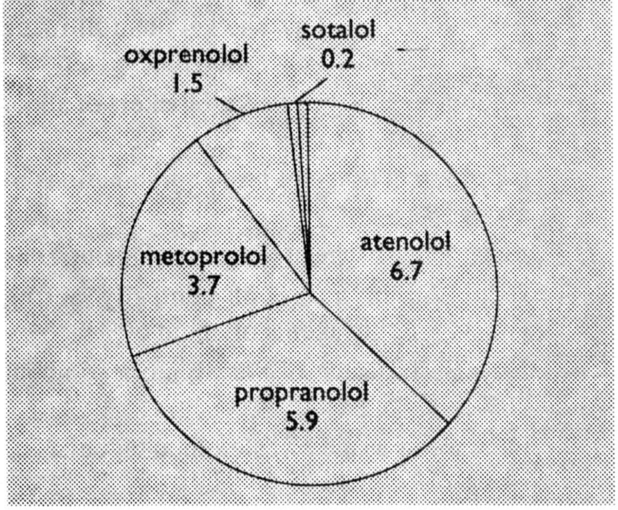

Fig. 5. Drug utilization study, Slovenia: a breakdown of individual fixed combinations prescribed (in DDD/1000 inhabitants/day)

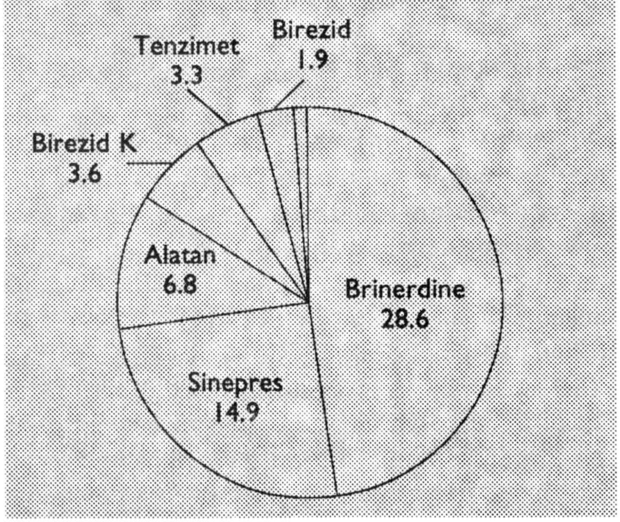

- increase in usage of ACE inhibitors (mainly enalapril) of about 145%.

The dynamics of drug utilization were influenced by various factors, such as:

- physicians' knowledge (education)
- patients' compliance
- the price of drugs (a factor of increasing importance)
- current information on the adverse and side effects of antihypertensive drugs.

The usage of antihypertensive drugs in Slovenia differs considerably from that in some other countries. A comparison with other centres is therefore of great interest.

The habit of prescribing several obsolete drugs is both persistent and deeply rooted. Replacement of the older generation of physicians with younger ones will hopefully result in better drug utilization.

Annex I

PROTOCOL FOR THE HYPERTENSION MANAGEMENT AUDIT PROJECT

1. Introduction

Hypertension has been repeatedly identified as a public health problem of worldwide dimensions and as one of the principal health problems of technically developed societies. The awareness of the great significance of hypertension has generated action in many countries, directed at the control of hypertension in the community. However, feedback information on changes of the earlier notoriously poor level of hypertension care is rather scanty. Special hypertension control projects have obviously been evaluated and their effectiveness has been demonstrated. However, the effects of programmes in selected communities or population groups are, expectedly, different from the impact of such action on the general level of detection and treatment of hypertension. There is information on trends in hypertension-related mortality (decreasing stroke and ischaemic heart disease death rates in certain countries), as well as drug prescription studies in selected areas, but this type of information, though very valuable, is related only to a few aspects of hypertension control.

The objectives of the project are, therefore, to produce information on the present status and quality of hypertension care.

2. Objectives

The project should be carried out in a number of centres in various countries. Inter-centre comparability of the findings is desirable; the protocol should be observed therefore as far as possible in all participating centres. However, local (national) situations may call for special considerations, allowing for a variety of optional inclusions, and the protocol may need to be adapted to the circumstances, resources and sources of information in a particular community.

The general aim of the study is to assess the level of hypertension control in various communities. The information to be obtained should be used for the improvement of hypertension control measures in the community.

Specific objectives are to assess:

(*a*) the level of awareness of hypertension in a community, by determining the proportion of undetected hypertensive subjects;

(*b*) the adequacy of care of known hypertensive subjects, including diagnostic work-up and possible under- or "over"-treatment;

(*c*) patients' acceptance of and satisfaction with the offered health care measures;

(*d*) physicians' knowledge and attitudes concerning the management of hypertension;

(*e*) the utilization of hypotensive drugs in a defined population.

Objective (*a*) necessitates a survey to determine the prevalence rates of known and unknown hypertension in the particular community (the community survey).

Objective (*b*) calls for a survey of known hypertensive patients (the patient survey).

Objective (*c*) can be approached by an inquiry into the opinions and attitudes of patients as consumers of health care (the consumer inquiry).

Objective (*d*) requires an inquiry into what physicians know and think about hypertension (the physician inquiry).

Objective (*e*) calls for a study of drug prescription and/or consumption (the drug utilization study).

Accordingly, the project consists of the following five parts: (*a*) community and (*b*) patient survey, (*c*) consumer and (*d*) physician inquiry, and (*e*) drug utilization study. Any of the five parts may be carried out independently, according to local possibilities and interest. Part (*a*), the community survey, is of fundamental importance, however, since any information from the other surveys or inquiries should be analysed in the context of the situation in the community. It is therefore suggested to carry out the community survey in any case, unless the appropriate information is available from other sources (e.g. MONICA survey).

3. Community Survey

3.1 Outline of procedures

The study design is outlined in Fig. 1. The subsequent steps are accompanied by estimates of numbers of subjects required or expected at each step. At least 3500 persons will be required at the outset, to ascertain sufficient numbers in further stages. The numbers indicated in Fig. 1 may be at the lower limit of acceptability.

3.2 Drawing of random sample

From a defined general population (e.g. electoral lists) a random sample should be drawn, including not fewer than 3500 subjects aged 35 – 64 years (both sexes). These age limits are set in order to streamline the project with MONICA. It is recommended, however, to include additionally the age group 65 – 74 years, in view of the great importance of hypertension in the elderly population.

Alternatively, a sufficiently big occupational group may be taken; this, however, will exclude subjects above 60 years (65 years) of age, though it would be desirable to obtain information on hypertension management in the elderly as well. Younger age groups may be included too, but will require a larger sample. Any characteristics of the population associated with hypertension should be described, e.g. high salt consumption or high prevalence of obesity.

3.3 Mailing invitation letter and basic questionnaire

Invitation letters should be drafted in each centre to suit the local style. The letter should explain the aims and importance of the study. If appropriate, the letter should be written in cooperation with the local medical society or physicians' association, or board of health. The basic questionnaire may be sent with the invitation letter or, alternatively, may be handed out when the subjects come to be examined.

Physicians and allied health workers of the area (community) should be aware of the study and their

Fig. 1. Outline of procedures for community survey and patient survey
(For description see text)

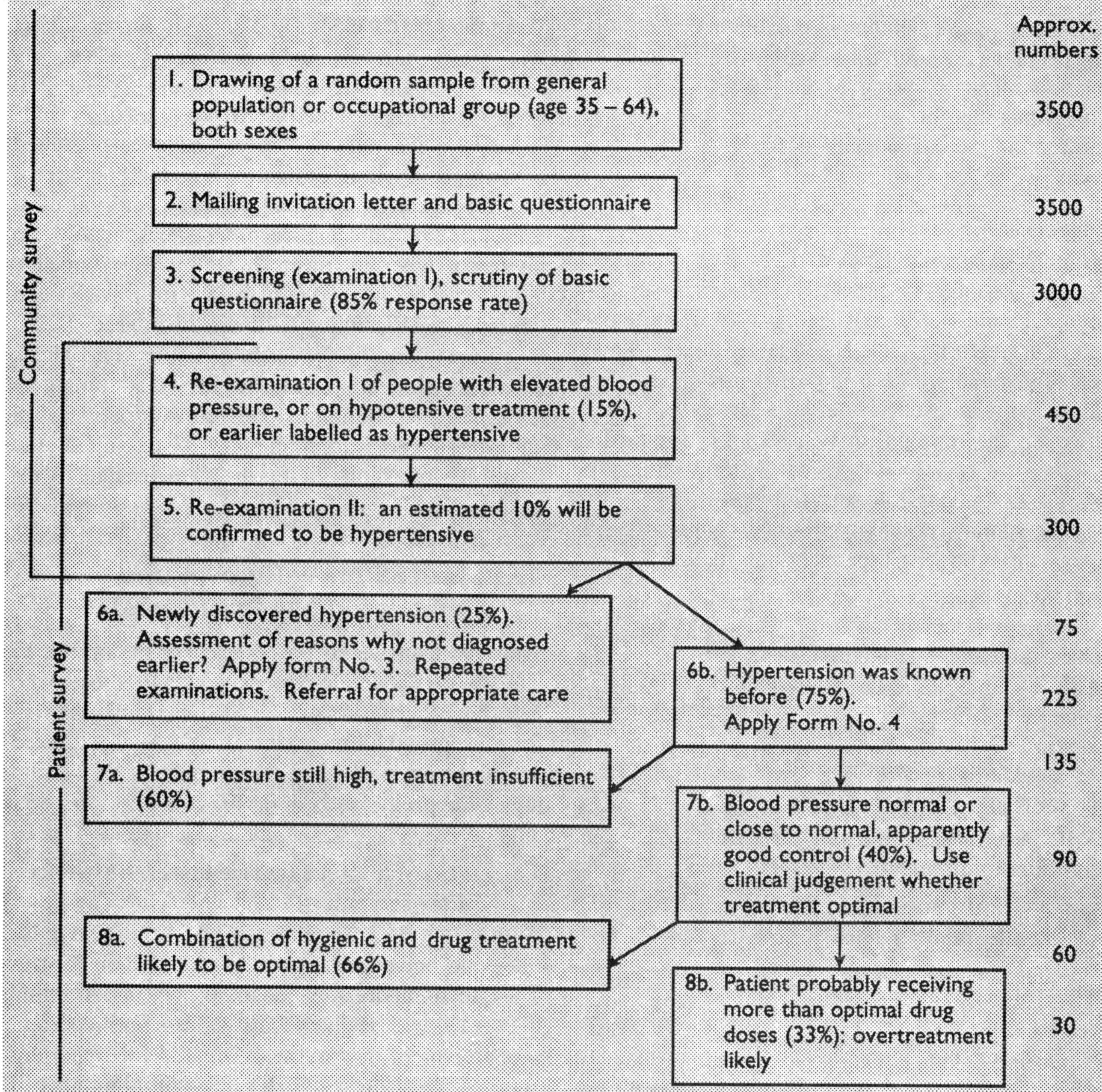

agreement and endorsement should be asked for. Involvement of and cooperation with primary health care physicians (GPs, district doctors, etc.) might become advisable, even unavoidable in certain settings, and the research team is reminded to consider the best means to achieve such cooperation. The whole approach hinges on the benevolent cooperation of the local physicians.

3.4 Screening (examination I)

With an expected response rate of 85%, some 3000 persons may be expected for the first (screening) examination. Should the response rate be below that figure, efforts should be made (reminders, home visits by social workers and other methods) to increase the response. Even at higher response rates, however, the reasons for non-response should be assessed by social workers or visiting nurses, in order to assess possible selection bias.

The social worker (or progress chaser) should clarify the following aspects of non-response:

1. Hypertensive status:	known treated known untreated
2. Blood pressure measured: (measure if possible)	never, last date value?
3. Any disease requiring medical care?	Yes, no
4. Disability, handicap, early retirement	
5. Occupation, educational grade, family status	
6. Declared reason for non-response.	

A reasonable timetable should be established for the screening examination, to avoid long waiting times and queueing upon arrival. The subject is greeted by a receptionist nurse or clerk who assists the screenee to complete the basic questionnaire or, if completed, checks it, and enters a serial subject number on Form 1. Then he/she proceeds to the measurement of BP [blood pressure], pulse and height and weight, which are all recorded on Form 1.

BP is measured preferably by a specially trained nurse or technician (see Section 5 on methods). Two BP measurements are made with an interval of at least three minutes and recorded. Persons with no history of hypertension and in whom at least one BP value was below 160 mmHg (S[ystolic] BP) and 95 mmHg (D[iastolic] BP), are dismissed as not meeting the criteria for further examination. Those with both values at or above either 160 mmHg or 95 mmHg will be invited for re-examination I. In addition, those who replied "yes" to any of the first three questions of Form 1 are invited to re-examination I.

4. Patient Survey (known and suspected hypertensives)

Those who answered "yes" to any of the first three questions (known hypertensives) and those who met the BP criteria (suspected hypertensives) will form the group for re-examination I. At an expected prevalence rate of 15%, the number of this group may be approximately 450.

4.1 Re-examination I (carried out 1 – 8 weeks after screening)

At this visit BP will be measured 3 times and pulse rate once, and all values will be recorded on Form 2. The questionnaire attached to Form 2 (or pertaining to Form 2) will be given to patients on antihypertensive treatment or previously treated for hypertension. (As it is foreseen that a substantial number of

Form 1

Basic questionnaire

Subject No. ☐☐☐☐☐

Family name -- Date ☐☐ ☐☐ ☐☐

First name -- Day Month Year

Sex: Male ☐ Female ☐

Year of birth ☐☐ Month ☐☐ Day ☐☐

Address: City ---------------------------- Street ---------------------------- No. ----------

Telephone No. ----------------

	Yes	No	Don't know
Have you ever been told that you have high blood pressure?	☐	☐	☐
If yes, have you ever been treated for high blood pressure?	☐	☐	☐
If yes, are you undergoing such treatment now?	☐	☐	☐

Please give names of drugs you take for hypertension:

Please give name and address of the physician you visit for your high blood pressure:

Do you agree that we may contact your physician for further information? ☐ Yes ☐ No ☐ Not applicable

Body weight ☐☐☐☐ kg

Height ☐☐☐☐ cm

Pulse rate ☐☐☐ b./min.

	Systolic	Diastolic	
Blood pressure I	☐☐☐	☐☐☐	mmHg
Blood pressure II	☐☐☐	☐☐☐	
Mean value of I and II	☐☐☐	☐☐☐	

Signature -- Place --

Form 2

Known and suspected hypertensives — re-examination I

Subject No. ☐☐☐☐☐

Family name .... Date ☐☐ ☐☐ ☐☐
Day Month Year

First name ....

Sex: Male ☐ Female ☐

Year of birth ☐☐ Month ☐☐ Day ☐☐

I. Systolic BP ☐☐☐ Diastolic BP ☐☐☐ Pulse rate ☐☐☐

II. Systolic BP ☐☐☐ Diastolic BP ☐☐☐

III. Systolic BP ☐☐☐ Diastolic BP ☐☐☐

Mean value ☐☐☐ Mean value ☐☐☐

individuals on antihypertensive treatment will decline the invitation to re-examination II, the importance of filling in the questionnaire at re-examination I is stressed.) (see Form 3). (The value of inviting all on antihypertensive treatment to re-examination II is recognized, but a substantial drop-out rate might be expected.)

4.2 Re-examination II (carried out 1 – 8 weeks after re-examination I)

All subjects who were eligible for re-examination I will be invited to re-examination II. It is expected that in about 10% of the originally surveyed population the diagnosis of hypertension will be confirmed. At this visit BP and pulse rate are measured three times and recorded on Form 2a.

In those with newly discovered hypertension, Form 3 is filled in and an assessment of the reasons why hypertension was not diagnosed earlier is made

4.3 Patients with previously known hypertension

Special efforts will be made to acquire all the earlier documentation available. Personal contacts should be established between senior project physicians and the patients' treating physicians (GP or specialist) or outpatient clinic. As a minimum, a random sample of at least 30 patients coming from at least five different doctors should be analysed.

The trend of thoughts as outlined in Fig. 1, 2 and 3 should be followed as much as possible. Form 4

Form 2a

Known and suspected hypertensives — re-examination II

Subject No. ☐☐☐☐☐

Family name ....

Date ☐☐ ☐☐ ☐☐
Day Month Year

First name ....

Sex: Male ☐ Female ☐

Year of birth ☐☐ Month ☐☐ Day ☐☐

I. Systolic BP	☐☐☐	Diastolic BP	☐☐☐	Pulse rate	☐☐☐
II. Systolic BP	☐☐☐	Diastolic BP	☐☐☐		
III. Systolic BP	☐☐☐	Diastolic BP	☐☐☐		
Mean value	☐☐☐	Mean value	☐☐☐		

will be completed with analytic care. The patients' history will be reconstituted by using information from the treating physician's documentation (patient file with its annexes) and all the information contained in the available study forms on the patient. Attention will be paid to such issues as side effects of drugs and their handicap, management by the treating physician of risk factors, psychological problems, work-site problems, etc.

The "reconstituted case" will be reviewed and reassessed by a task force of three physicians, which will include at least one senior physician, preferably the principal investigator.

The quality of hypertension care will be assessed. Overtreatment is considered an interesting point, though such a conclusion may be based on a value judgement. Overtreatment may exist when blood pressure presumably would be still acceptable either (1) without drug therapy, or (2) with lower doses, or (3) with fewer drugs, or (4) with milder drugs (preparations causing fewer side effects). To this may be added (5) the possibility of using less expensive drugs.

When considering whether drug administration has been optimal, the patient's treatment history should be scrutinized.

Overtreatment can be stated with certainty only if drug therapy has been changed and the effects of the change observed. Since this usually may not be feasible, overtreatment mostly remains a statement on a probability or possibility.

When there is no indication that treatment with lowest doses and fewest drugs has been attempted, this may be taken as a strong hint that overtreatment has possibly occurred.

Form 3

Patient survey: assessment of reasons why hypertension was not diagnosed earlier

Subject No. ☐☐☐☐☐ Date ☐☐ Day ☐☐ Month ☐☐ Year

When was subject medically examined for the last time? ☐☐ Day ☐☐ Month ☐☐ Year

What kind of examination was it?

	Acute disease	*Chronic disease*	*Injury*	*Unknown*	*None*
General practitioner	☐	☐	☐	☐	☐
Specialist	☐	☐	☐	☐	☐
Hospital	☐	☐	☐	☐	☐
Home visit	☐	☐	☐	☐	☐
Occupational (factory)	☐	☐	☐	☐	☐
Unknown	☐	☐	☐	☐	☐

	Yes	*No*		*Yes*	*No*
Invited for health examination[a]	☐	☐	Attended	☐	☐

	Yes	*No*	*Does not remember*
Was blood pressure measured at that examination?	☐	☐	☐
Was subject told anything about the blood pressure values?	☐	☐	☐
If yes, was it elevated?	☐	☐	☐
normal?	☐	☐	☐
no clear statement?	☐	☐	☐

Subject's interpretation why his hypertension has not been discovered earlier (use subject's own wording, as far as possible)

....

....

Examiner's interpretation why hypertension has not been discovered earlier

....

....

[a] Includes examinations such as periodic visits, check-ups without disease, screening visits, fluoroscopy, examinations for driver's licence, employment, etc.

Fig. 2. The patient survey: assessment of diagnosis (for policlinics, outpatient departments, etc.)

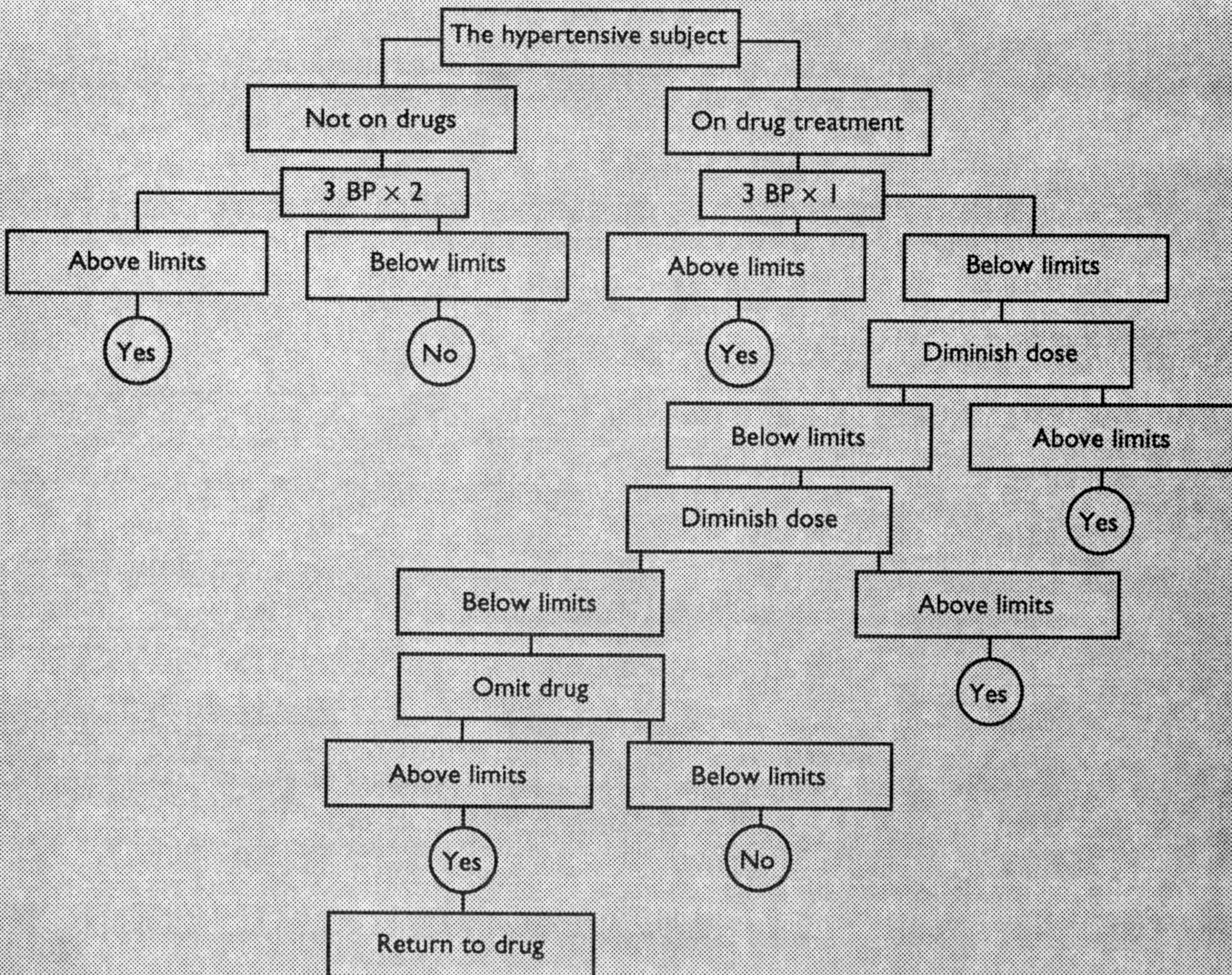

Note. Limits refer to Bürgenstock recommendations [*Bulletin of the World Health Organization*, **61**: 53 – 56 (1983).]

Hypertensive subject: any patient diagnosed previously as hypertensive, whether or not on treatment.

3 BP × 2: three blood pressure readings on two occasions (separate visits); average value of the six readings.

(Yes) hypertension confirmed.

(No) hypertension not confirmed.

Fig. 3. The patient survey: assessment of treatment

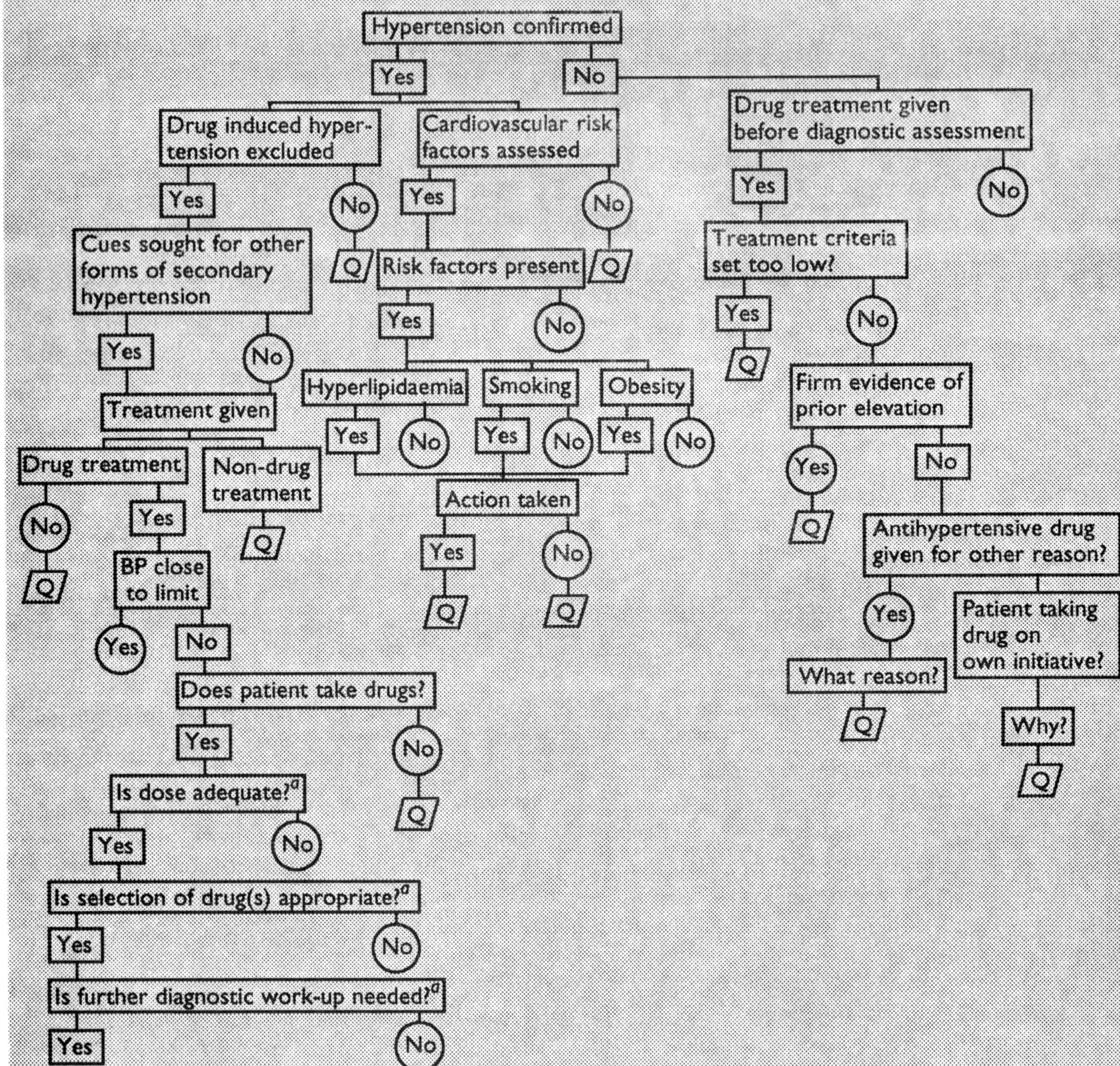

[a] Standards of WHO Hypertension Manual refer.

Note. Q Ask questions about reasons (apply questionnaire).

Clinical judgement will be applied with circumspection, especially for classification into 7a and 8a/8b. If no consensus is reached within the task force, an outside resource person should be consulted.

5. Blood Pressure Methods in Community and Patient Survey

5.1 Blood pressure measurement

Measurements of blood pressure are best carried out by the indirect method, using a mercury sphygmomanometer. The patient should be seated comfortably in a quiet room. The arm muscles should be relaxed and the forearm supported. A cuff of suitable size is applied evenly and firmly to the exposed upper arm. Care should be taken to avoid tight sleeves. The cuff width for an average-sized adult should be 13 – 15 cm. Larger cuffs are needed for patients with fat arms [. . .]. The cuff should be inflated while the radial or brachial pulse is felt, until the pulse disappears. This point gives the approximate systolic pressure.

The cuff is then reinflated and slowly deflated, during which time the Korotkoff sounds are heard through a stethoscope placed over the brachial artery. The pressure at which the sounds are first heard is the systolic pressure [. . .]. The diastolic pressure (phase V) is the pressure at which the sound disappears. Most of the major studies have used the latter point, which may be significantly lower than the phase IV pressure. Because most of the data concerning treatment have been related to phase V diastolic pressure, this should be used when deciding on the need for treatment.[a]

The systolic and diastolic pressures should be measured at least twice with at least three minutes between. At the screening examination the lowest reading is recorded; at subsequent re-examinations the mean value of the two measurements is taken into account.

5.2 Training for blood pressure measurement

Blood pressures are preferably measured by specially trained nurses or technicians. Training may be done by special teaching tapes or films, or by careful direct tuition. For details, see Rose & Blackburn, *Cardiovascular survey methods*, 1981.[b] Frequent quality control, including digit preference, should be performed.

Legend and comments to Fig. 2

Fig. 2 and Fig. 3 expand in more detail the patient survey procedures summarized in the lower part of Fig. 1. They give a flow chart of the trend of thoughts to be followed by the task force (review committee) which is carrying out the patient survey. Fig. 2 shows how to assess the validity of the diagnosis of arterial hypertension in persons in whom hypertension was diagnosed previously. The aim is to find possible cases of overdiagnosis.

The hypertensive subject is any patient diagnosed previously as hypertensive, regardless of whether he is or is not on drug treatment at the time of the survey. If the subject is not on drug treatment, three blood pressures are taken on two re-examinations made at

[a] Guidelines for the treatment of mild hypertension: memorandum from a WHO/ISH meeting. *Bulletin of the World Health Organization*, **61**: 53 – 56 (1983).

[b] Rose, G.A. & Blackburn, H. *Cardiovascular survey methods*. Geneva, World Health Organization, 1981 (Monograph Series, No. 56).

an interval of approximately seven days. If the mean value of the six measurements is above 140/90 mmHg, the diagnosis of hypertension is confirmed. If the mean value of the six measurements is below 140/90 mmHg, the diagnosis of hypertension is *not* confirmed.

If the patient is on drug treatment, three blood pressures are taken on the first re-examination and the mean value calculated. If the mean value is above the limits of 140/90 mmHg, the diagnosis of hypertension is confirmed. If the mean value of blood pressures is below these limits, the dose of the drug should be diminished. The patient then should be re-examined after one to three weeks. If the mean value of three blood pressures is now above the limits, the diagnosis of hypertension *is* confirmed. On the other hand, if blood pressure is still below the limits, the same procedure should be repeated as shown on the flow chart. Finally, if when omitting the drug the patient's blood pressure is still below the limits, the diagnosis of hypertension is *not* confirmed; on the other hand, if blood pressure rises above the limits when the drug had been omitted, the diagnosis *is* confirmed and the patient should return to drug treatment.

Legend and comments to Fig. 3

This figure gives detailed guidelines of the trends of thought when analysing the previous treatment of a hypertensive subject.

If the diagnosis of hypertension has not been confirmed as described in Fig. 2, and drug treatment was given to the patient, the question should be asked by the task force whether the treatment criteria were set too low during the previous treatment of the patient. If this was not the case, the patient either might have had firm evidence of blood pressure elevation in the past, or antihypertensive drugs might have been given for some other reasons (e.g. diuretics or beta-blockers) or the patient might have been taking drugs on his own initiative. It is desirable to ask for the reasons in any of these cases.

The left-hand part of the flow chart refers to cases in which the diagnosis of hypertension *has* been confirmed. The trend of thoughts follows two branches; the right-hand branch shows what kind of questions should be asked concerning other cardiovascular risk factors possibly associated with high blood pressure. One should also ask questions about action taken in the presence of risk factors such as hyperlipidaemia, smoking or obesity. If no action was taken, one should ask why. If action *was* taken one should ask whether it was appropriate and effective.

The left-hand branch describes the reasoning concerning drug treatment. It takes into account whether the possibility of drug-induced hypertension was excluded, whether thought has been given to other forms of secondary hypertension and whether treatment was given. The considerations of secondary hypertension do not necessarily include elaborate diagnostic procedures such as pyelography, renography, etc.; it only refers to the question whether the possibility of secondary hypertension had been considered at all.

As regards treatment, consideration should be given to non-drug treatment and to drug treatment. If the patient is on drug treatment and his pressure is still far from reaching the desired values, the question should be asked whether he is in fact taking the prescribed dose or not. If the patient is not complying with the prescribed therapy one should try to find the reasons for it. If, on the other hand, the patient does take the prescribed drugs, the question should be asked whether the choice of the drug(s) was appropriate, whether the prescribed dose is adequate or whether any further diagnostic work-up is needed.

In order to facilitate the analysis, two further forms are proposed; the key questions to be asked in the patient survey are formalized on these record forms. However, they may need to be adapted to the local situation (Forms 3 and 4).

6. The Consumer Inquiry

The consumer inquiry may be done independently or linked with the patient survey. This part of the project applies to patients with diagnosed hypertension. As pointed out earlier, the objectives are to assess the patients' satisfaction or criticism of the health care they are receiving. The purpose of the inquiry is possibly to eliminate the reason for the discontent of the patients, assuming that such improvement will contribute to the strengthening of hypertension control in the respective community. The patient inquiry must be tailored to the local situation in the community and take into consideration the local culture. Therefore the patient inquiry form is only a model that should be adapted and, if possible, expanded (Form 5).

The questionnaire may be filled in by an interviewer, or may be handed out as a self-administered questionnaire.

According to the local situation and interest of the investigator, various practical questions should be asked as well, for example referring to waiting time, friendliness or unpleasant attitude of health personnel, difficulties of reaching the centre because of problems in city transportation, availability or lack of parking space around the centre, queueing, cleanliness of premises, including toilets (where applicable), etc. Also, the patients should express their opinion concerning the physicians, the time they are devoting to their patients, and their ability to listen and to explain. If felt desirable, the questionnaire should be made anonymous. This again depends on the local situation.

7. The Physician Inquiry

The objective of the physician inquiry is to obtain insight into the knowledge and attitudes of physicians in the community concerning the management and treatment of hypertension. It is assumed that if the weaknesses in the physician's knowledge and attitudes can be defined, the control of hypertension in the community could be improved by addressing targeted information to the medical corps in the particular community.

The physician inquiry can be carried out independently of the other parts of the project. Nevertheless, it is useful to make it in conjunction with the other components of the project.

The general practitioners and internists working in the area should be included into this project. A sample size of approximately 300 physicians is considered appropriate. If there are more of them in the area, a random sample may be selected. If their number does not exceed much the requirement for this study, all of them may be included. If the community has fewer than 300 physicians, all of them should be included.

A self-administered questionnaire should be sent out to general practitioners (primary health care physicians) and internists working outside the hospitals. The questionnaire should be simple enough and its completion should not take more than 10 – 15 minutes. It has to be accompanied by a covering letter, tactfully inviting the physicians to participate in the inquiry and informing them on the advantages they may derive from the project (Form 6).

Although it would be important to assess the actual behaviour of the physicians instead of their attitudes, this would be too difficult to achieve and could lead to tensions and to the antagonizing of the medical profession in the area. It may be assumed, however, that the actual practice of the physicians is

Form 4

Patient survey: assessment of work-up and treatment in patients with previously diagnosed hypertension

Subject No. ☐☐☐☐☐ Date ☐☐ ☐☐ ☐☐ (Day Month Year)

HEALTH WORKER IN CHARGE OF PATIENT

None = 0	General practitioner = 2	Other physician = 4
Specialist = 1	Occupational physician = 3	Nurse = 5

Total observation period: Years ☐☐ Months ☐☐

Observation period before drug treatment was started: Years ☐☐ Months ☐☐

How many blood pressure measurements were taken before treatment was started? ☐☐

How many of these blood pressure readings were at or above 160 and/or 95? ☐☐

	Yes	*No*	*Unknown*
Was family history taken?	☐	☐	☐
Was body weight measured?	☐	☐	☐
Was height measured?	☐	☐	☐
Was a urine analysis done?	☐	☐	☐
Was an ECG taken?	☐	☐	☐
Was a serum potassium performed?	☐	☐	☐
Was a serum creatinine done?	☐	☐	☐
Was a serum cholesterol done?	☐	☐	☐
Was a serum uric acid done?	☐	☐	☐
Was a post-load blood sugar done?	☐	☐	☐
Was a chest X-ray taken?	☐	☐	☐
Was eye-ground examination done?	☐	☐	☐
Other diagnostic procedures performed?	☐	☐	☐

Which? ....

....

Form 4 (contd)

Is smoking habit of patient recorded? ☐☐☐

Is alcohol intake recorded? ☐☐☐

Is use of oral contraceptives recorded? ☐☐☐

How many visits did the patient have during the first year? ☐☐

How many visits did the patient have during the last year? ☐☐

Record the last 3 BPs taken

1. Systolic ☐☐☐	2. Systolic ☐☐☐	3. Systolic ☐☐☐
Diastolic ☐☐☐	Diastolic ☐☐☐	Diastolic ☐☐☐

TREATMENT

	Yes	*No*	*Unknown*	*Not applicable*
Was patient found to be overweight?	☐	☐	☐	☐
Was any non-pharmacological treatment instituted?	☐	☐	☐	☐
If *yes*, what type: Weight reduction?	☐	☐	☐	☐
Sodium restriction?	☐	☐	☐	☐
Physical exercise?	☐	☐	☐	☐
Other?	☐	☐	☐	☐

If drug treatment is given presently, what drugs?

Name and dose

..................................Beta-blockers		☐	☐	☐
..................................Diuretics		☐	☐	☐
..................................Vasodilators		☐	☐	☐
..................................Rauwolfia		☐	☐	☐
..................................Calcium antagonists		☐	☐	☐
..................................Centrally acting sympathicolytic drugs		☐	☐	☐
..................................Others		☐	☐	☐

TASK FORCE CONCLUSION

Patient belongs to category 7a ☐ 8a ☐ 8b ☐ (see Fig. 1)

Form 5

Consumer inquiry: known and suspected hypertensives

Subject No. ☐☐☐☐☐

Date ☐☐ ☐☐ ☐☐
Day Month Year

OPTIONAL: MAY BE FILLED IN ANONYMOUSLY

Family name --

First name --

Sex: Male ☐ Female ☐

Year of birth ☐☐ Month ☐☐ Day ☐☐

Address: City ------------------------ Street ------------------------ No. --------

Telephone No. ------------

1. Is it difficult to be a patient with high blood pressure? No = 0 Yes = 1 Hard to say = 2 ☐

2. How satisfied are you with the care given previously for your high blood pressure?
   Very satisifed = 1
   Satisfied = 2
   Not satisfied = 3
   Very dissatisfied = 4
   No opinion = 5 ☐

3. When was the last time you took drugs for high blood pressure?
   Today or yesterday = 1
   2 – 3 days ago = 2
   One week ago = 3
   One week to one month ago = 4
   More than one month ago = 5
   Other, when = 6 ☐

4. Do you take your drugs for high blood pressure regularly? No = 0 Yes = 1 ☐

5. When visiting a clinic, is it important for you to meet the same doctor? Nurse?
   Absolutely = 1
   Rather = 2
   Not especially = 3
   Not at all = 4
   No opinion = 5 ☐

Form 5 (contd)

6. Do you usually see the same doctor?	Always = 1 Often = 2 Seldom = 3 Never = 4 Do not know = 5	☐
7. Occasional deviations in drug taking are quite common. On average, how often during the last month have you missed your tablets (or some of them)?	Never = 1 Once or twice in the last month = 2 Once a week = 3 Several times a week = 4 Nearly every day = 5	☐
8. Do you think that it is easy to remember to take the tablets as prescribed?	No = 0 Yes = 1	☐

unlikely to be better than the views and attitudes reflected in the replies to the questionnaire.

As in the other parts of the project, the proposed questionnaire may be adapted to the local situation.

8. Drug Utilization Study

This is a useful complement to the other parts of the study. It may be carried out on its own. If such a study is taking place independently of the present Hypertension Management Audit Project, efforts should be made to establish links between the two projects and to exchange information related to hypertension.

8.1 Methodology

The ATC (Anatomical-Therapeutic-Chemical) classification and the defined daily dose (DDD) should be used. The ATC classification has been published, together with guidelines for its use, by the Nordic Council on Medicines and is the method followed by the WHO Drug Utilization Research Group (DURG). Copies of this publication are available from the Nordic Council on Medicines.

8.2 Measurements

Measurements should be in defined daily doses (DDD) per 1000 inhabitants per day. DDDs have been established for many of the single component drugs by the WHO Collaborating Centre for Drug Statistics Methodology in Oslo. For drugs to be monitored which do not yet have DDDs assigned to them, individual centres should establish the DDDs in consultation with the WHO Collaborating Centre.

8.3 List of drugs to be monitored

(*a*) Beta-blockers (monosubstance preparation)

(*b*) Beta-blockers in combination with another drug, diuretics or other combination

(*c*) Diuretics

(*d*) Diuretics combined with sympathicolytics (reserpine, ergot alkaloids)

Form 6

Physician inquiry questionnaire

Name (optional) -- Date ☐☐ ☐☐ ☐☐
Day Month Year

Age ☐☐ years Sex M ☐ F ☐

General practioner ☐ Internist ☐ Cardiologist ☐ Other ☐ (CHECK ONE)

A . BLOOD PRESSURE MEASUREMENT IN THE OFFICE

1. Who is measuring BP in your office?
   - nurse ☐
   - physician ☐
   - physician assistant ☐

2. How do you measure BP in a patient?
   - right arm ☐
   - left arm ☐
   - both arms ☐
   - sitting position ☐
   - lying position ☐
   - standing position ☐

3. How long is the interval between repeated BP measurements? ☐

4. What BP measurement device do you use in your office?
   - Mercury sphygmomanometer ☐
   - Automatic device ☐
     - If yes, what kind (company name) --
   - Aneroid BP device ☐

Form 6 (contd)

5. How often do you standardize your BP measurement devices?
   - once a year ☐
   - once in 2 years ☐
   - less frequently ☐

6. What cuff sizes do you use in adult patients?
   Give width and length of cuff bladder --

7. What Korotkoff sounds do you use for DBP measurements?
   - Korotkoff IV ☐
   - Korotkoff V ☐

8. Do you record BP values to the nearest 10 mmHg? ☐
   5 mmHg? ☐
   2 mmHg? ☐

9. Do you think patients' self-measurement of BP is useful? Yes ☐ No ☐
   Do you teach your patients self-measurements? Yes ☐ No ☐

10. When has your *own* BP last been checked? Month ☐☐ Year ☐☐

B. HANDLING OF PATIENTS IN THE OFFICE

1. How many patients overall did you see in your practice last year? ☐☐☐
2. How many hypertensive patients did you have in your practice last year? ☐☐☐
3. Do you keep a register of hypertensive patients in your practice? Yes ☐ No ☐
4. Do you use a reminder system for your hypertensive patients? Yes ☐ No ☐
5. Do you actively invite your hypertensive patients for control? Yes ☐ No ☐
6. Do you think that a computer in your office could help you in setting up a reminder system for your hypertensive patients? Yes ☐ No ☐

Form 6 (contd)

C. ATTITUDES TOWARDS HYPERTENSION CONTROL

1. What BP values do you consider hypertensive?

age: below 35	systolic BP	☐☐☐
35 – 59	systolic BP	☐☐☐
60 and above	systolic BP	☐☐☐
below 35	diastolic BP	☐☐☐
35 – 59	diastolic BP	☐☐☐
60 and above	diastolic BP	☐☐☐

2. At what BP values do you consider drug treatment essential?

age: below 35	systolic BP	☐☐☐
35 – 59	systolic BP	☐☐☐
60 and above	systolic BP	☐☐☐
below 35	diastolic BP	☐☐☐
35 – 59	diastolic BP	☐☐☐
60 and above	diastolic BP	☐☐☐

3. Do you apply non-drug treatment in your hypertensive patients? If yes, what type?

Weight reduction	Yes ☐	No ☐
Sodium restriction	Yes ☐	No ☐
Physical exercise	Yes ☐	No ☐
Behavioural therapy	Yes ☐	No ☐
Stopping oral contraception	Yes ☐	No ☐
Other	Yes ☐	No ☐

4. Do you inquire about other cardiovascular risk factors?

Smoking	☐
Hyperlipidaemia	☐
Alcohol	☐

Form 6 (contd)

D. DIAGNOSTIC PROCEDURES

1. Which of the following procedures do you perform for the diagnostic work-up of your hypertensive patients?

Body weight measurement	Yes ☐	No ☐
Height measurement	Yes ☐	No ☐
Urine analysis	Yes ☐	No ☐
ECG	Yes ☐	No ☐
Serum potassium	Yes ☐	No ☐
Serum creatinine	Yes ☐	No ☐
Serum cholesterol	Yes ☐	No ☐
Serum uric acid	Yes ☐	No ☐
Post-load blood sugar	Yes ☐	No ☐
Chest X-ray	Yes ☐	No ☐
Eye-ground	Yes ☐	No ☐

E. THERAPEUTIC PROCEDURES

1. What is your first choice of antihypertensive drugs as monotherapy?

	Males	*Females*
age: below 35	☐	☐
35 – 59	☐	☐
60 and above	☐	☐

List of drugs:

Beta-blockers	☐
Diuretics	☐
Vasodilators	☐
Rauwolfia	☐
Calcium antagonists	☐
Others	☐

2. Do you reduce the dose of antihypertensive drugs after normalization of your patient's BP?

Yes ☐ No ☐

Form 6 (contd)

F. ATTITUDES

1. Do you think that the activities concerning hypertension control in the media are sufficient?

Television	Yes ☐	No ☐
Radio	Yes ☐	No ☐
Newspaper	Yes ☐	No ☐

2. Do you think that information on hypertension via the media supports the physician's treatment of hypertensive patients?

   Yes ☐ No ☐

3. Do you think that continuous medication has negative psychological effects in your hypertensive patients?

   Yes ☐ No ☐

4. Do you think that side effects of antihypertensive drugs must be accepted or tolerated by the patients?

   Yes ☐ No ☐

G. HOW DO YOU USUALLY OBTAIN INFORMATION ON HYPERTENSION AND OTHER CARDIOVASCULAR RISK FACTORS?

a) Medical journals ☐
b) Continuous education programmes ☐
c) Textbooks ☐
d) Pharmaceutical industry information ☐
e) Television/radio/newspapers ☐
f) Leagues against hypertension ☐
g) WHO ☐
h) ISH ☐
i) National high blood pressure education programme ☐

(*e*) Diuretics combined with vasodilators and other components

(*f*) Synthetic hypotensives and other

(*g*) Calcium antagonists.

The WHO Collaborating Centre on Drug Statistics Methodology prepared a detailed list following the ATC classification, with a listing of the DDDs where these exist. For combination drugs, centres should formulate their own proposals in consultation with the WHO Collaborating Centre on Drug Statistics Methodology.

8.4 Sources of data

(*a*) *Statistics*

- wholesale statistics (Intercontinental Medical Statistics)
- diagnosis index (Intercontinental Medical Statistics)
- hospital drug use (Ministry of Health, National Health Board hospitals)
- reimbursed drugs (social/health insurance)
- pharmacies.

(*b*) *Prescriptions – social or health insurance and/or pharmacies*

- continuous sample (1/288)[a]
- all prescriptions, several cross-sectional (1 month/year)
- ad hoc studies
- individual-based monitoring continuous follow-up
- pharmacies.

Wholesale data should be collected to measure the intensity of medication in the population, and the prescription data should be used as the means of interpreting the data thus collected, with regard to age and sex distribution.

Physician and patient sources were also considered, but the group felt that the data obtained would be too soft to be of use. Individual centres may wish, however, to collect the information in a standardized way from these sources, and proposals for questionnaires are being prepared for the final report.

8.5 Data collection in individual centres

Each centre planning drug monitoring should describe its proposals for data collection, as well as plans for validating the data collected, and send these to the WHO Collaborating Centre for review and comment. For drugs on the international market for which DDDs exist, this form of measurement should be used. For drugs with no established DDD, the measurement should be decided between the WHO Collaborating Centre in Norway and the individual centres.

Address of the WHO Collaborating Centre for Drug Statistics Methodology in Oslo:

Dr K. Øydvin
Norsk Medicinaldepot
Postbox 100 Veitvet
Oslo 5
Norway.

[a] Represents number of working days per year.

Annex 2

PHYSICIAN INQUIRY IN THURINGIA, GERMANY

G.M. Pfaff, German Institute for Hypertension Research, Heidelberg, Germany & G. Stein, Clinic for Internal Medicine, Friedrich-Schiller-University, Jena, Germany

A physician inquiry was carried out in a sample of general practitioners and internists in the former district of Gera, German Democratic Republic. This area, situated close to the geographical centre of Germany and now part of the federal state of Thuringia, has about 730 000 inhabitants. One third of its population live in the cities of Gera (134 500) and Jena (107 500). The area is adjacent to the former district of Erfurt where a reporting unit for the MONICA project is located.

The objective was to obtain information from physicians who had been involved in primary care for hypertensive patients in the former German Democratic Republic. While physician inquiries had been conducted in cities in western Germany (see Chapters 13 and 14), no corresponding data had been collected for the former German Democratic Republic.

Methods

The sample consisted of general practitioners and internists who were members of two medical societies for general and internal medicine incorporated in the German Democratic Republic prior to its accession to the Federal Republic of Germany in October 1990. Physicians were eligible if they were residing or working in the former district of Gera and involved in primary medical care at the time of the survey. The study was performed over a nine-week period between March and May 1991. Physicians received a self-administered questionnaire, together with a stamped return envelope. Wherever possible, the wording of questions was kept identical to the surveys conducted earlier in western Germany, except where they needed to be adjusted to differences in the structure of the health care system in eastern Germany. Non-respondents received a reminder letter five weeks after the first mailing. Owing to local conditions, no telephone contacts were sought.

Results

Among the 367 addressees, 38 (10%) were identified as not meeting the criteria for eligibility (other medical specialties, not in primary care, no longer in study area, retired, deceased). Of the remaining 329 physicians, 221 (67%) returned a valid questionnaire (162 general practitioners and 59 internists).

Of these, 35 respondents (16%) (including 33 internists) worked in hospitals with outpatient clinics. Among the physicians working in facilities giving outpatient care exclusively, about 50% were in private practice, with the rest working in ambulatory clinics or rural dispensaries. Ages ranged from 29 to 84 years (still in practice), with a mean of 48 years.

Table 1 lists the reasons for measuring blood pressure in patients seen. One in two physicians indicated that they checked blood pressure routinely in all patients.

Table 2 summarizes the techniques of blood pressure measurement used. In 57% of primary health care institutions, mercury sphygmomanometers were used exclusively; in most others, mercury devices were used alternately with other systems. Measurements on the right arm were preferred, with 10% of physicians conducting measurements on both arms. One in two institutions standardized blood pressure devices at intervals of two years or less, as required by legislation in the former German Democratic Republic. Korotkoff phase V was used by 81% of respondents.

Table 3 reflects the blood pressure levels at which drug treatment was considered essential. In general, physicians in Thuringia were more inclined to initiate drug therapy in systolic hypertension, and showed more restraint in diastolic hypertension.

In the work-up of newly diagnosed hypertensive patients, an average of 11 diagnostic procedures was considered essential. As shown in Table 4, urine analysis, weight, total cholesterol, serum creatinine and electrocardiogram recording were quoted by more than 90% of respondents.

Among the non-drug measures advised for the treatment of hypertension in Table 5, attention was most often paid to weight reduction. At the same time, 83% of the responding physicians estimated that fewer than 10% of their hypertensive patients were treated exclusively with non-drug measures.

The first choice of drugs in the treatment of newly diagnosed hypertensive patients are shown in Table 6. Preferences varied according to the age group of patients but were independent of the patients' sex.

Table 7 shows that, when blood pressure control has been achieved, about one third of all physicians

Table 1. Physician inquiry, Thuringia: reasons for measuring blood pressure

Reason	Percentage of physicians
Done routinely	47
Patient is known hypertensive	88
Done for every new patient	65
Patient has special complaints	68
Hypertension is suspected	71
Hypotension is suspected	67
Done once every year in all patients	25

Table 2. Physician inquiry, Thuringia: reported practices in blood pressure measurement

Reported practices	Percentage of physicians
Measurement taken:	
by physician	96
by nurse	62
Measurement taken:	
on right arm	36
on left arm	18
on both arms	10
it varies	35
Routine measurement:	
in sitting position	81
in supine position	5
in various positions	15
Frequency of blood pressure measurement during one consultation	
only once	34
twice	59
three times	6
Device used	
mercury only	57
aneroid only	3
automatic only	4
more than one	34
Different cuff sizes applied	
no	73
yes	6
sometimes	20
Device standardized:	
once a year	14
once in two years	29
less often	56
Sounds used	
Korotkoff V	81
Korotkoff IV	17
Rate of decrease of pressure during measurement	
10 mmHg per second	6
5 mmHg per second	31
2 mmHg per second	19
not pre-set	39
Physician's own blood pressure checked during current or last calendar year	83

Table 3. Physician inquiry, Thuringia: level of blood pressure values at which physicians consider drug treatment essential

Blood pressure (mmHg)	Percentage of physicians
Systolic	
< 140	0
140 – 149	2
150 – 159	17
160 – 169	57
170 – 179	15
≥ 180	9
Diastolic	
< 90	0
90 – 94	6
95 – 99	29
100 – 104	53
≥ 105	12

Table 4. Physician inquiry, Thuringia: diagnostic procedures always performed by physicians

Procedure	Percentage of physicians
Body weight	92
Height	62
Urine analysis	98
Electrocardiogram	97
Serum potassium	59
Serum creatinine	95
Total cholesterol	94
Serum uric acid	63
Fasting blood sugar	86
Post-load blood sugar	7
Chest X-ray	84
Eye-ground examination	81

Table 5. Physician inquiry, Thuringia: non-drug measures advised

Measure advised	Percentage of physicians
Body weight reduction	99
Sodium restriction	81
Physical activity	82
Healthy nutrition	80
Smoking intervention	75
Exercises for relaxation, stress reduction	23
Other	11

Table 6. Physician inquiry, Thuringia: physicians' first choice drugs for newly initiated antihypertensive treatment, by age and sex of patient

First choice drug	Percentage of physicians who choose drug in patients aged:		
	< 35 years	35 – 60 years	60 + years
In male patients			
Beta-blockers	88	40	6
Diuretics	15	28	41
Vasodilators	4	22	25
ACE inhibitors	8	31	41
Calcium antagonists	14	57	66
Others	0	2	2
In female patients			
Beta-blockers	81	39	5
Diuretics	16	29	39
Vasodilators	6	23	27
ACE inhibitors	7	27	38
Calcium antagonists	14	53	63
Others	0	3	2

Note. Figures for individual age and sex groups do not add up to 100% as multiple responses were permissible.

Table 7. Physician inquiry, Thuringia: changes in drug dosage after reduction of blood pressure

Action	Percentage of physicians
Reduce dosage	35
Sometimes reduce dosage	54
Make no changes	10
No response	1

reduced the drug dosage. In addition, one in two physicians indicated that they reduce drug dosage occasionally.

In summary, the replies of this group of physicians from the eastern part of Germany reflected generally adequate attitudes and opinions about the diagnosis and management of hypertension, comparable to those in other parts of Europe. While systematic blood pressure checks for all patients seen in the physician's office need to be propagated more intensely, the diagnostic work-up of identified hypertensives appears to be thorough. Some overuse of diagnostic procedures, such as chest X-rays, seems to occur similarly to other centres. Compared with earlier inquiries in western German cities (see Chapter 13), the preference for Korotkoff phase V was higher among physicians in Thuringia than among western German colleagues who might have been influenced by an earlier controversy about the use of phase IV measurements.

These physicians seem to exert more restraint in starting drug treatment than their colleagues in the western parts of Germany. Such a conservative attitude may have been caused by the previously limited selection of available drug categories. Another possible explanation could be less exposure in the past to messages recommending the initiation of drug therapy at lower blood pressure levels. The indicated drug preferences in the treatment of newly diagnosed hypertension show a high acceptance of the new classes of antihypertensive drug that had become widely available in the 18 months preceding the inquiry.

The accession of the former German Democratic Republic to the Federal Republic of Germany in October 1990 resulted in structural changes to the primary health care system; outpatient care was transferred from clinics and dispensaries with or without hospital affiliation to newly founded private practices. The data therefore illustrate the management of hypertension in a health care system in transition.

Annex 3

PRELIMINARY RESULTS FROM INDIA

S. Padmavati, Director, National Heart Institute and President, All India Heart Foundation, New Delhi, India

The present project began in June 1989. Three centres, representative of north, central and southern India, were selected at Delhi, Nagpur and Coimbatore. At each centre, the investigators chosen were consultant physicians interested in hypertension and familiar with epidemiological work. They also had contacts with local general practitioners and other physicians, because of their good professional standing.

Nagpur later withdrew from the project and at present only two centres, Delhi and Coimbatore, are carrying out the work.

Two approaches were taken, the community survey and the physician inquiry. While the community survey results are complete for both Delhi and Coimbatore, the physician inquiry results from Coimbatore are not yet finalized. Only the Delhi results are therefore presented.

Community Survey

The prevalence of hypertension was low in both centres, lowest in Coimbatore (Table 1). Awareness of hypertension was also low (Table 2).

Table 1. Community survey, Delhi and Coimbatore: prevalence of hypertension

Centre	No. of subjects		Number (%) of hypertensives			
			First examination		Second examination	
	Male	Female	Male	Female	Male	Female
Delhi	3020	980	120 (3.973)	43 (4.387)	115 (3.8)	40 (4.08)
Coimbatore	3000	400	24 (0.8)	4 (1)	20 (0.66)	3 (0.75)

Table 2. Community survey, Delhi and Coimbatore: awareness and treatment status of hypertensives

Centre	Number (%) of hypertensives:		
	aware of hypertension	under treatment	
		Male	Female
Delhi	78 (50)	60 (50)	20 (50)
Coimbatore	18 (78)	15 (75)	3 (100)

Main characteristics of the sample

Of 155 individuals studied in Delhi, most were aged between 41 and 60 years. Most cases of hypertension were mild, with diastolic blood pressure values of 90 – 95 mmHg. Obesity was seen in 10%, most were vegetarians, smoking was seen in 10% (none of them women) and alcohol consumption in only 3%. Of the laboratory data, blood sugar levels suggestive of diabetes were seen in 20%, none of whom were aware of this. Serum cholesterol levels were normal in the majority. Serum triglycerides were raised in only a small number (11%) in whom diabetes was also present (Table 3).

Treatment

Because of difficult access to medical care, only 80 out of 155 patients received regular treatment. As they were not symptomatic, they did not seek medical attention from their general practitioners. A higher proportion of patients received treatment at Coimbatore because of easier access to medical care. None of the patients had measured their own blood pressure, but those who were under treatment had gone to their local practitioners for blood pressure measurement.

Physician Inquiry

For this inquiry, 76 general practitioners who were reputed to have a large practice and were in the age group 45 – 60 years were sent a questionnaire based on the protocol (Annex 1) and received a phone call about filling it in; 50 returned the questionnaire (a response rate of 66%). There was considerable delay in receiving replies from some of these practitioners, and a social worker had to be sent to help them fill out the answers. These physicians all have the basic qualifications of MBBS and no postgraduate qualifications. They attend refresher courses organized by the local medical associations. A similar questionnaire has been mailed to 20 cardiologists and 30 internists (general physicians) who have postgraduate qualifications beside the MBBS. Their answers have been received only in part and will be compiled when complete.

The replies (Table 4) show that the physicians measure blood pressure as there are no nurses in most general practitioners' surgeries in India. Most of the measurements were done in the sitting position. The interval between the repeated measurements was five minutes. Mercury sphygmomanometers were used by 30 physicians and aneroid devices by 20. Standardization was unsatisfactory. No answers were given

Table 3. Community survey, Delhi: main characteristics of sample

Characteristic	Male	Female	Total	(%)
Sample size	115	40	155	(100)
Age (years)				
< 40			56	(36.1)
41 – 60			62	(40)
60 +			37	(23.9)
Degree of hypertension				
mild			120	(77.41)
moderate			30	(19.35)
severe			5	(3.24)
Obesity (over 20% body weight)	10	6	16	(10)
Smoking (over 2 packs/day)	16	0	16	(10)
Alcohol consumption (over 60 g/day)	5	0	5	(3.2)
Diet				
vegetarian			120	
nonvegetarian			35	
Blood sugar level				
normal (< 120 mg)			93	(60)
borderline (130 – 150 mg)			31	(20)
high (> 180 mg)			31	(20)
Serum cholesterol				
normal (< 200 mg)			109	(70.32)
borderline (200 – 240 mg)			46	(29.68)
Serum triglycerides				
< 150 mg			119	(76.8)
151 – 200 mg			19	(12.2)
> 240 mg			17	(11.0)

Table 4. Physician inquiry, Delhi: summary of questionnaire results

Date: Jan 1990 – June 1991

Age: 45 – 60 years

Sex M [40] F [10]

General practitioner [50] Internist [✓] Cardiologist [✓] Other [ ] (CHECK ONE)

A. BLOOD PRESSURE MEASUREMENT IN THE OFFICE

1. Who is measuring BP in your office?	
nurse	0
physician	50
physician assistant	0
2. How do you measure BP in a patient?	
right arm	35
left arm	15
both arms	0
sitting position	45
lying position	5
standing position	0
3. How long is the interval between repeated BP measurements?	5
4. What BP measurement device do you use in your office?	
Mercury sphygmomanometer	30
Automatic device	
If yes, what kind (company name) ------------------------------	
Aneroid BP device	20

Table 4 (contd)

5. How often do you standardize your BP measurement devices?
   - once a year [0]
   - once in 2 years [3]
   - less frequently [47]

6. What cuff sizes do you use in adult patients?
   Give width and length of cuff bladder --

7. What Korotkoff sounds do you use for DBP measurements?
   - Korotkoff IV [30]
   - Korotkoff V [20]

8. Do you record BP values to the nearest 10 mmHg? [0]
   - 5 mmHg? [10]
   - 2 mmHg? [40]

9. Do you think patients' self-measurement of BP is useful? Yes [30] No [20]
   Do you teach your patients self-measurements? Yes [ ] No [✓]

10. When has your *own* BP last been checked? Month [|] Year [|]

B. HANDLING OF PATIENTS IN THE OFFICE

1. How many patients overall did you see in your practice last year? [3|0|0|0] (mean)
2. How many hypertensive patients did you have in your practice last year? [|6|0]
3. Do you keep a register of hypertensive patients in your practice? Yes [5] No [45]
4. Do you use a reminder system for your hypertensive patients? Yes [2] No [48]
5. Do you actively invite your hypertensive patients for control? Yes [ ] No [✓]
6. Do you think that a computer in your office could help you in setting up a reminder system for your hypertensive patients? Yes [ ] No [✓]

Table 4 (contd)

C. Attitudes towards hypertension control

1. What BP values do you consider hypertensive?

age:	below 35	systolic BP	140
	35 – 59	systolic BP	150
	60 and above	systolic BP	160
	below 35	diastolic BP	90
	35 – 59	diastolic BP	95
	60 and above	diastolic BP	

2. At what BP values do you consider drug treatment essential?

age:	below 35	systolic BP	150
	35 – 59	systolic BP	160
	60 and above	systolic BP	
	below 35	diastolic BP	90
	35 – 59	diastolic BP	95
	60 and above	diastolic BP	

3. Do you apply non-drug treatment in your hypertensive patients? If *yes*, what type?

	Yes	No
Weight reduction	40	
Sodium restriction	50	
Physical exercise	45	
Yoga and meditation	20	
Stopping oral contraception	–	
Other (alcohol)	5	

4. Do you inquire about other cardiovascular risk factors?

Smoking	Yes
Hyperlipidaemia	Yes
Alcohol	Yes

Table 4 (contd)

D. Diagnostic procedures

1. Which of the following procedures do you perform for the diagnostic work-up of your hypertensive patients?

Body weight measurement	Yes	50	No	
Height measurement	Yes		No	
Urine analysis	Yes	50	No	
ECG	Yes	40	No	
Serum potassium	Yes		No	
Serum creatinine	Yes	30	No	
Serum cholesterol	Yes	45	No	
Serum uric acid	Yes	–	No	
Post-load blood sugar (random)	Yes	30	No	
Chest X-ray	Yes	25	No	
Eye-ground	Yes	–	No	

E. Therapeutic procedures

1. What is your first choice of antihypertensive drugs as monotherapy?

age	*Males*	*Females*
below 35	–	–
35 – 59	–	–
60 and above	–	–

List of drugs	
Beta-blockers	25
Diuretics	30
Vasodilators	
Rauwolfia	45
Calcium antagonists	20
Others (ACE inhibitors)	15

2. Do you reduce the dose of antihypertensive drugs after normalization of your patient's BP?

Yes 2 No 48

Table 4 (contd)

F. Attitudes

1. Do you think that the activities concerning hypertension control in the media are sufficient?

Television	Yes		No	50
Radio	Yes		No	50
Newspaper	Yes	20	No	30

2. Do you think that information on hypertension via the media supports the physician's treatment of hypertensive patients?

Yes 50 No

3. Do you think that continuous medication has negative psychological effects in your hypertensive patients?

Yes – No –

4. Do you think that side effects of antihypertensive drugs must be accepted or tolerated by the patients?

Yes 15 No 35

G. How do you usually obtain information on hypertension and other cardiovascular risk factors?

a) Medical journals	25
b) Continuous education programmes	24
c) Textbooks	10
d) Pharmaceutical industry information	48
e) Television/radio/newspapers	5
f) Leagues against hypertension	
g) WHO	
h) ISH	
i) National high blood pressure education programme (All India Heart Foundation)	15

about cuff sizes. The majority still use the Korotkoff sound phase IV. Blood pressure was measured to the nearest 2 mmHg. The majority were in favour of the self-measurement of blood pressure. There was no satisfactory answer as to whether they measured their own blood pressure. Very few kept a register of hypertensive patients or sent reminders. The answers about the use of computers were negative.

The majority considered a blood pressure level of 140/90 mmHg high in patients under 35 years of age and 150/95 mmHg as hypertensive in patients aged between 35 and 59 years.

With regard to the level when drug treatment should start, this was pretty low compared to many other studies reported. Non-drug treatment of hypertensive patients was familiar to general practitioners and the value of salt restriction, weight reduction and physical exercise was well known. There was no reply about oral contraceptives. Yoga and meditation are very much a part of the Indian ethos and were recognized as a means of controlling hypertension. All the general practitioners were aware that smoking, hyperlipidaemia and alcohol could worsen the effects of hypertension. Diagnostic procedures included urine analysis, electrocardiogram, serum cholesterol, blood sugar (random) and chest X-ray. This shows a good knowledge of investigative procedures.

With regard to therapeutic procedures, no distinctions were made between older and younger age groups. With regard to the first choice drugs, rauwolfia came first, followed by diuretics, beta-blockers, calcium antagonists and ACE inhibitors in that order. Rauwolfia was first introduced to the world from India and a favourite prescription is Adelphane Esidrex, which contains hydralazine and rauwolfia. None of the physicians reduced the drugs when the blood pressure level came down. Most of the physicians considered the media unsatisfactory in projecting hypertension control measures.

The side effects of antihypertensive drugs were well known, but were expected to be tolerated by patients if they wished to attain effective blood pressure control.

The main source of information on hypertension was the pharmaceutical industry; 50% obtained this information from medical journals and continuing medical education programmes, and 30% from the All India Heart Foundation publications.